Text, illustrations, and photography copyright© 2015 by Mollie Walker Freeman. All rights reserved. No part of this book may be reproduced or transmitted in any form, or by any means, electronic or mechanical, including photocopying, recording, or by any information storage or retrieval system without written permission of the publisher, except as permitted by law.

Mail requests to: Permissions, Big Picture Publishing, 185 Harrison Avenue, Loveland, Colorado 80537. email: Mollie@LifeSongNutrition.com

Special thanks to Scott W Freeman and Benjamin McMillan

Library of Congress Catalog-in-Publication-Data
Freeman, Mollie Walker. Eating Bugs - A Fermentation Sensation! / by Mollie Walker Freeman; illustrations and photographs by Mollie Walker Freeman; design by Benjamin McMillan
p. cm. Summary: This book explains why and how to culture or ferment foods, and provides recipes to culture foods at home.

Printed in the United States of America

ISBN 987-0-9906097-3-5

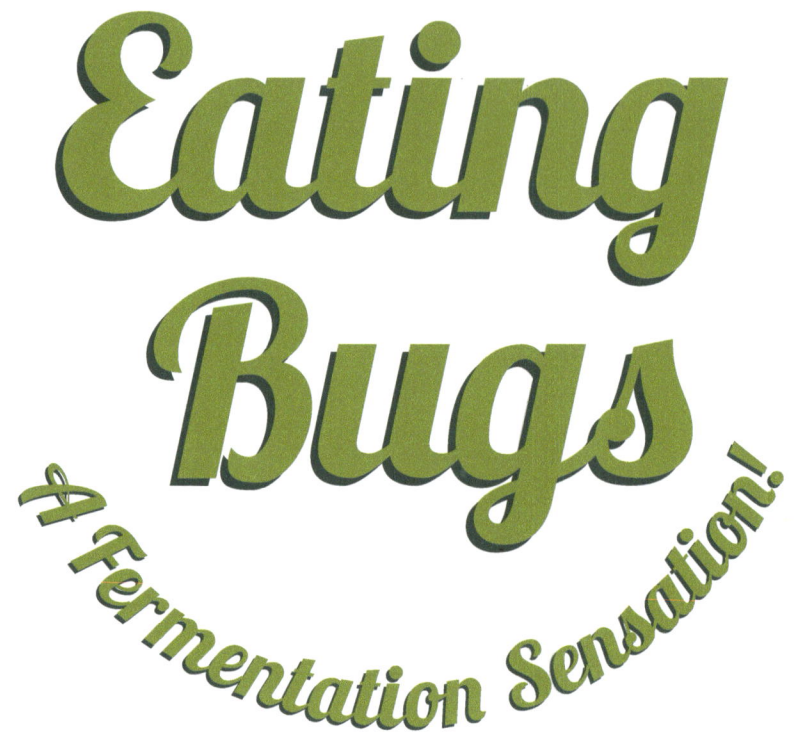

By Mollie Walker Freeman

Certified Health Coach

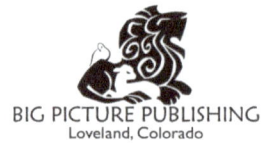

BIG PICTURE PUBLISHING
Loveland, Colorado

Table of Contents

Part 1 - What's so great about fermentation?

- 6 What You'll Find Here
- 9 Your Internal Environment
- 11 Good Guys And Bad Guys
- 12 My Own Story
- 13 Bug Balancing Act
- 14 Cultured Foods Help Real People Heal
- 16 What Fermentation Does To Foods
- 17 Detoxification

Part 2 - How Can I Do This At Home?

22 **Inoculating Your Ferment**

Veggies To Ferment

- 26 Pepper Kraut
- 28 Japanese-Style Sauerkraut
- 30 Cranberry Citrus Ferment

32 Warming Winter Beets

34 Zucchini And Onions

36 Italian-Style Tomatoes

38 Autumn Spaghetti Squash

Cultured Fruit Recipes

42 Berries And Pears

44 Lemons With Goji

46 Mango Peach Ferment

Beverages

49 Kombucha

56 Flavors

58 Green Veggie Juice With Green Tea

60 Ginger Ale

Condiments

64 Easy Cultured Mustard

66 Mango Salsa

68 Lacto Fermented Ketchup

Sourdough

72 Sourdough Pancakes

74 Yam Muffins

76 Cultured Oatmeal

78 **A Word About Cultured Dairy**

What You'll Find Here

In this book, let's see what's so great about fermented foods and the bugs that make them so phenomenal. We'll take a look at what people are saying about how cultured foods have helped them to heal from digestive distress, skin problems, fibromyalgia, and more. But I'll also give you some great recipes and instructions so you can begin to prepare these foods yourself. If you're watching your food budget, you'll be happy to know that it's extremely economical to incorporate these foods. And if your schedule is already too full, I'll point you in the right direction so you can find some awesome cultured products to purchase.

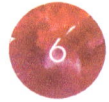

Part 1:
What's so great about fermentation?

Do you want to have more energy and less discomfort after eating? Are you bothered by poor elimination, headaches, interrupted sleep, especially with late night eating? Are you battling mysterious symptoms? Skin problems? Autoimmune disorders? Are you trying to get most of your nutrition from your foods (instead of from pills), while knowing that our depleted soils, food storage and transportation issues, and processing, and a host of other factors have rendered our foods much less nutrient dense than they should be?

      Cultured and fermented foods are almost magical, in my estimation. They have the potential to transform your body by re-building your digestive micro-flora. Believe it or not, all of the aforementioned health concerns (and more!) can be helped – and in some cases, cured – by incorporating these foods into the diet. Cultured foods are loaded with vitamins and micro-nutrients which multiply during the fermentation process. At the same time, there is such a wide variety of processes and flavors of these wonder foods that your menus can also be transformed for the better! It's not just about yogurt and sauerkraut (though these can be a great start). It all starts with bacteria – the friendly kind! – to which I often refer as "bugs."

Your Internal Environment

Who wants to hear about creepy crawlies that take up residence in or on the human body? I, for one, had about all I could stomach with seeing a film of the tiny mites that inhabit all of our eyelashes. Somehow it makes the subject it a little more approachable for me to know that I never have to actually see the critters that live in my gut—all 100 trillion of them! As Jennifer Ackerman of Scientific American puts it,"Bacteria cells in the body outnumber human cells by a factor of 10 to 1."

The great news is that most of these bacteria are, in fact, friendly. They are actually some of our greatest internal allies. The not-so-great news is that many of us have inadvertently killed off large numbers of these friendly bacteria. Did you have a lot of ear infections as a child? Perhaps one or two really major illnesses for which you were given antibiotics? Did you ever have a yeast infection? What about stress? Ever have that??? Maybe you've eaten more than the recommended 6 teaspoons of sugar per day (American Heart Association's recommendation). Maybe sugar is not your thing, but you eat fast food, or a lot of processed foods. Or perhaps you know you have some food allergies or sensitivities. Maybe you just don't eat many vegetables (except for ketchup!), or perhaps you don't really drink water (coffee & bottled juice are good enough, right?)

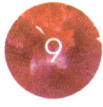

As if all these challenges are not enough, we now see from the latest research that glyphosate, the world's most common pesticide also has a very detrimental effect on our healthy gut bacteria. While we have been assured that this chemical, which turns up in soil and water samples all over, and also in blood samples from animals & people, has no adverse effect on humans, we now know that this is only part of the picture. Glyphosate works by interrupting a metabolic pathway in plants called the "shikamate pathway." While humans do not have this pathway, micro-organisms that live in humans do have it! When you remember that, head to toe, 90% of the cells in you, by number, is actually microbiota, you can see the problem easily. So, eating commercially raised plant foods, especially corn and soy products, which are nearly all treated with glyphosate, is also a risk factor for compromised gut health.

Good Guys And Bad Guys

If any of the risk factors above ring true for you, you may not have nearly as many friendly bugs as you need. I think of this microbial picture a bit like an army—two opposing armies, really. I'm sure this is over-simplified, but bear with me. So, you have the "good guys" and the "bad guys." If all goes according to design, you are born with some good guys, which quickly multiply into a good army while you are still an infant. Breast feeding helps to nourish your army. If you then are invaded by bad guys, your good army will fight them off. And really, I should say, "when you are invaded," because germs and invaders come regularly. As long as your good army of beneficial bacteria are intact and you immune system is otherwise functioning properly, you can fend off or recover from these various attacks. In fact, as I understand it, your good guys continue to increase and your immune system is strengthened.

My Own Story

What happened in my own gut as a baby was different. Since my mother is no longer living, it was tough to piece together all the details, but as near as I could figure, she did not breast feed me for very long—a few weeks, probably. At the age of 3 months, I nearly died from pneumonia. I was hospitalized and given massive amounts of antibiotics. I am thankful, of course, that I came out of all that alive! Antibiotics killed the harmful bacteria in my body. Unfortunately, they also killed the "good guys."

I subsequently had numerous ear & throat infections throughout childhood, followed by several yeast infections as a teenager. I do not remember a time when my digestion or elimination was good. I would be about 40 years old before I would learn about the missing friendly bugs in my gut. Now, the balance of bacteria in the body is always in flux, but mine just never seemed to strike a healthy balance

Bug Balancing Act

When the balance of bacteria is not what it should be in a person's intestinal tract, harmful bacteria can multiply out of control. At the same time, other factors may be causing inflammation and damaging the friendly micro-flora. This includes things like eating lots of sugar and/or processed foods, or eating foods to which one is sensitive or intolerant. If you want to learn more about this process, look up "leaky gut" on the internet.

There is so much to know about this topic that I will leave it to you, because this book is not about what leaky gut is; it's about what you can do to right the balance of friendly gut flora, heal your intestines, dramatically improve your digestion, and enjoy your life more than ever! Once your digestion is optimized, you will experience increased energy and vitality; and you will not have to endure the gas, bloating, elimination issues, and general discomfort associated with low levels of healthy gut flora. In addition, you will be able to assimilate all those good nutrients you take in; so all the cells of every system in your body will be able to improve in function (assuming, of course, that you are consuming lots of nutritious foods.)

Cultured Foods Help Real People Heal

For years, I've heard about the amazing healing properties of lacto-fermented foods. I'm absolutely certain they have played an important role in my own healing, though I suppose there may be no way to prove that claim. I have also heard other health coaches talk about how they recommend fermented foods to their clients with excellent results.

The health claims I've heard associated with these foods comprise a very long (and ever increasing) list. Remember, the process of lacto-fermentation is said to increase levels of B vitamins & folic acid, vitamin C, Omega-3 fatty acids, and helpful enzymes which help to digest lactose and proteins. So, it's not hard to imagine that eating them would improve immune system function, reduce inflammation, and calm symptoms of an irritable bowel. Auto-immune disorders are said to improve as a result of the consumption of cultured foods, too. Rheumatoid arthritis, Multiple Sclerosis, Addison's disease, and Celiac are mentioned on the website MindBodyGreen.com as being positively responsive to the addition of fermented foods to the diet and healing the gut.

Since fermented foods benefit the gut, naturally, digestive problems can be diminished or eliminated with help from our "good bug" friends. But here's another exciting benefit: another eliminative organ is also benefitted. Do you think of your skin this way? The skin helps your body get rid of toxins, and can become overloaded in today's environment. Fermented foods lighten the load

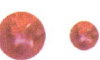

of the skin while also nourishing it to reportedly clear up acne, eczema, psoriasis, and other skin problems in many cases.

      According to DoctorOz.com, eating cultured foods can also help with weight management by contributing to stable blood sugar. Another reported benefit is mental clarity. This is not hard to believe either when you consider that much of your serotonin can be found – you guessed it – in your gut. A great website, FireflyKitchens.com, asserts that lacto-fermented foods promote healthy blood pressure and cholesterol levels. While you're on the web, check out Cindy Sparling's story at FibromyalgiaTreatmentGroup.com. This site makes a strong connection between systemic inflammation and auto-immune disorders, such as fibromyalgia. They also recommend dietary suggestions to heal naturally, including fermented foods.

What Fermentation Does to Foods

Any bacteria, given the right conditions, will multiply rapidly. And surprisingly, helpful bacteria are already hanging out all over the place, on the surfaces of plants and animals, and even on your own skin! During the fermentation process, we encourage the proliferation of good bacteria, which will, in turn, inhibit the growth of harmful bacteria. (Think of the army analogy again.) But what happens to the food as it cultures is truly amazing!

First of all, the process or fermenting multiplies and "unlocks" nutrients, making them much more bio-available. This means that all those micro-nutrients are ready to be used by your body's cells. Some authors use the term "pre-digested" to describe what happens here. So, if you have had trouble with the assimilation of nutrients, like I have, eating cultured foods can help. See Genkifoods.com for more on this.

As the vegetables, fruits, milk, (or whatever food you use) cultures, lactic-acid bacteria is being produced. This is why you will sometimes see the term "lacto-fermentation." The term has nothing to do with lactose, which is milk sugar. If you are vegan or dairy intolerant, you need not avoid lacto-fermented foods! A good explanation of this can be found at pickl-it.com.

Detoxification

It is important to note that your body's response to cultured foods is individual. If you normally eat lots of processed foods or are unaccustomed to eating this type of fermented foods (as opposed to foods pickled using vinegar), you may need to introduce cultured foods gradually. Start with a teaspoon or so each day, and after a week or so, add another teaspoon. Eventually, you will be able to consume a quarter to half a cup per day of fermented fruits and vegetables, as well as kombucha, kefir or yogurt and others. If you feel discomfort when you eat too many of these foods at first, it is probably because a bit of a detoxification response is occurring in your body.

Especially if you are also adding in other nutrient dense foods, such as green vegetables, and dramatically reducing processed foods, sugar, or other items which have been troubling you, you may feel some discomfort or fatigue associated with your body's natural inclination to cleanse itself of toxins. Simply slow down the transformation process a little. It is also a good idea to seek the advice or supervision of a health professional. Do not be discouraged! Cultured foods will ultimately help and can produce nearly miraculous results. I have heard about a few individuals who say they are too sensitive for cultured foods, and cannot eat them. If you feel, at any point, that you are experiencing a bad reaction to these foods, seek the advice of a professional. I personally have not seen such a case, however.

It is worth noting here that consuming organic produce and grains whenever possible will lighten your toxic load. I recommend using the highest quality foods in every recipe, but I do not specify "organic" for individual items. Using locally produced foods tends to be advantageous, as well, in terms of nutrient value as well as flavor. This is partly because of minimal transit and storage.

Part 2:
How Can I Do This At Home?

I'm going to start you out with some simple basics, but once you get the knack, you'll be able to make all sorts of recipes easily. Since vegetables are the easiest and least likely to go wrong in any way, let's talk about them first. There are several techniques for making a ferment happen in your kitchen. Some involve special equipment like earthenware crocks or special weights for holding the vegetables under the liquid during the process.

The essential things for making fermented veggies include: the veggies themselves, a glass or earthenware container with a lid, and either salt, brine (from a previous batch), whey, some other source of good bacteria, or a combination of these. You'll also need to have some sort of liquid that will cover the veggies, as mentioned above. This might be filtered water or freshly made juice of some kind, or it may be simply juice from the items you are fermenting. The first natural sauerkraut recipe I read, many years ago, called for beating the cabbage with a hammer to release the juice of the cabbage!

It is important to note that in using the techniques I teach, the produce must be submerged during the fermentation process. (There are other techniques that are anaerobic, sealing the fermenting items off from air. They work in a slightly different way.) If parts of it are protruding above the liquid, they will be subject to mold. You can usually avoid mold by either taking measures to keep your produce submerged, or by stirring and poking it back down every day. I have had success with some recipes by tightly closing the jar lid and not touching it for up to a few weeks.

At other times, I have used the "open air" method. In this technique, the produce is submerged under plenty of liquid, but the lid is left off of the container so that the bacteria from the environment can access the ferment. In this method, it is a good idea to weight down the produce to keep it from floating up to the surface and molding. I have used a glass filled half way with water, at times. My favorite weight is a smooth rock that fits nicely into my jar mouths. I took care to thoroughly wash it first, of course, and I also boiled it for several minutes in water on the stove top. Once the veggies are secured, I cover the whole thing with a dish towel to keep dust and dog hair out.

Another important thing to note is that heat destroys bacteria. During the culturing process, temperature is important. Generally, the ideal temperature for fermentation to occur is about room temperature, 68 – 72 degrees Fahrenheit. If the foods are heated enough to cook, the culturing process is stopped. When we make cultured baked goods, the fermentation happens prior to baking, and is very beneficial. However, there are no live micro-organisms in the finished product. If you desire to consume the healthful bacteria, you will want to add your fermented items (such as sauerkraut or cultured salsa) to foods just prior to eating them – not during the cooking process.

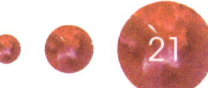

Inoculating Your Ferment

It is possible to ferment vegetables without any "starter" culture. Remember that the friendly bacteria are already on the veggies? By liberally salting the veggies, the harmful bacteria are suppressed long enough for the good bugs to grow. That said, I really am not fond of that much salt (though a small amount is fine). Also, the recipes that allow for using salt only (and no starter) seem to call for a longer period of fermentation. I have tried using this method a few times, with success, but I do not prefer it.

What I like to use more often than not is liquid whey. According to Sarah Pope, Chapter leader in the Weston A. Price Foundation, powdered whey will not work in this process. However, until I saw her video on YouTube, it never occurred to me to try the powdered form. Extracting the whey is simple, and takes only a few minutes to set up, provided you have a plain cotton tea towel or several layers of cheese cloth. Simply place about a cup of plain yogurt or kefir into the center of the cloth, gather up the sides of the cloth and fasten with a tie or rubber band, then hang up over a bowl. The whey will drip out into the bowl during the next couple of hours. What is left in the cloth is a wonderful cultured cream cheese. I like to add a little salt to it and my daughter spreads it on carrots or crackers. Now you have whey for fermenting!
If you do not have whey, and if you do have a previous batch of fermented veggies which are similar in flavor to the new batch you want to create, you can strain off a few tablespoons of brine to use as a starter instead of the whey.

You can also share brine with a friend!

There are a couple of ways of mixing the items for the recipes. One way is to stuff chopped veggies into a jar or crock, pushing them down forcefully with a wooden spoon or your fist, salting layers lightly every inch or so. This can make a very pretty package if you are using a clear jar and colorful ingredients in layers. When you have filled the jar with your produce, you can add the liquid. Just make sure you leave at least an inch of space at the top, as the ferment will expand a bit during the process.

The other way to do it is to chop your produce with a knife and place it into a large bowl. (You could also use a food processor to chop it.) When the various ingredients are in the bowl, you can easily salt and mix them all together. This is a good method to use if you are making a large batch of any recipe. Again, push the veggies into your jars or crocks; cover with water, juice, or a mixture of the two. Last, add brine (from a previous batch) or whey.

If you are at all sensitive to molds, I recommend using the anaerobic method with air lock seals, which can be found at Pickl-it.com.

Next: a few recipes to get you going!

Veggie Recipes to Ferment

Pepper Kraut

Shredded cabbage, about 75% of the volume of your jar or crock

Chopped bell peppers (any color), about 15 - 20%

Chopped onion (any color), about 5 – 10%

Hot peppers (jalapeno or habanero) – small amount, optional

This is a perfect thing to make in early fall when the garden is overflowing with peppers and cabbage. Onions are not hard to come by either. Simply push down all the ingredients into your crock or jar, sprinkling with salt after every inch or two is packed in. Then, top with your water and whey or brine from a previous batch. If you don't have anything with which to inoculate this culture, just make sure you use about 2 teaspoons of salt for a quart jar. Keep out of direct sunlight. I like to cover mine with a dark towel or place inside a cabinet.

You'll want to let this recipe culture at about 70 degrees Fahrenheit for about 2-3 weeks. I have said "about" because there are several factors which cause the length of time to vary. If your temperature gets much above 71 or 72 degrees, the fermentation could happen very quickly. In fact, you are in danger of spoilage in that case, and I recommend finding a cooler place to keep it. If, on the other hand, it is cool in the spot where you have your culture working, say 68 degrees or below, it could take twice as long to get a nice flavor. Also, it depends upon the flavor you personally prefer. I like to taste my kraut every day or two after the first week, and put it into the fridge when it's pleasantly tangy.

If your produce does, in fact, spoil, you will know it! Sauerkraut has a bit of a stinky smell (in my opinion) even when it's good. But if it spoils, which happens rarely, it will be intolerably bad. If you open the jar and find a white film, do not panic! This is a friendly, probiotic yeast. If you find mold or evidence of other invaders, it's safest to throw out this batch.

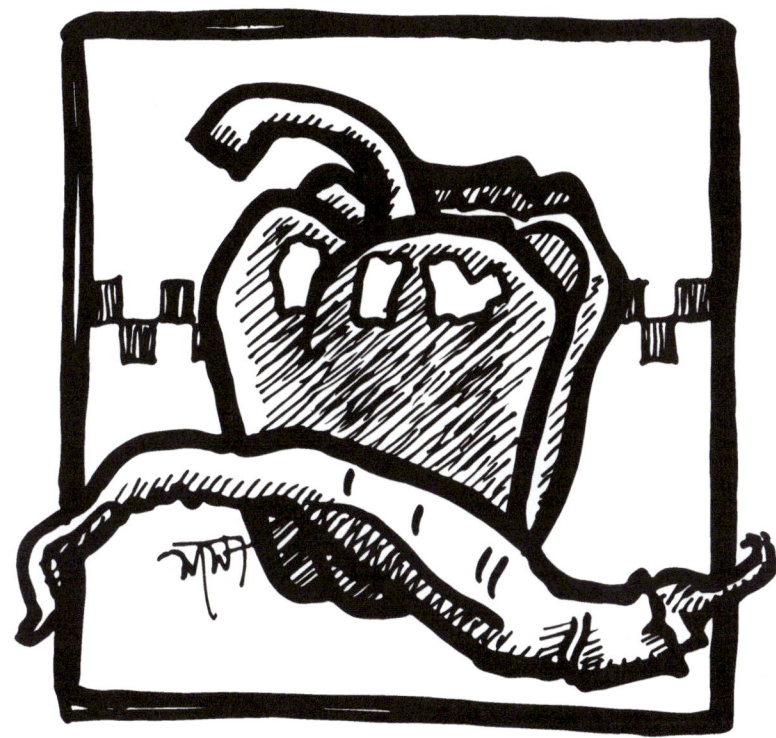

Japanese-Style Sauerkraut

Napa or Savoy cabbage, shredded, about 75% of the volume of your container

Diakon radish, sliced or matchstick cut, about 10%

Carrot, shredded, about 10%

Green onion, chopped, about 5%

Ginger root, shredded, to taste

Mustard seeds, whole, 1-2 teaspoons per quart

Poppy seeds, 1-2 teaspoons per quart

½ teaspoon miso, mixed thoroughly with ¼ cup water – use this amount for a quart recipe

I like to toss all of these ingredients, except for the miso/water, in a large bowl, then stuff them into a jar. I then prepare the miso and water, and pour it over the top of it all. The last thing I will do is add a teaspoon of brine from a previous batch, if I have it, and top with more water. Miso is fermented, so it not only adds a nice, salty flavor, but it also inoculates your sauerkraut. You can find miso at a natural foods grocery or an Asian food store. Leave at least an inch of empty space at the top of your container to allow for expansion.

Sometimes this recipe tastes fabulous after only a few days. It does not smell great, however. Don't be put off by the smell of any sauerkraut! You have to get past the sulfur odor and taste it in order to appreciate this phenomenon. I have read recipes for sauerkraut that call for much longer fermentation. Feel free to experiment or scan the internet for different opinions & ideas!cause the length of time to vary. If your temperature gets much above 71 or 72 degrees, the fermentation could happen very quickly. In fact, you are in danger of spoilage in that case, and I recommend finding a cooler place to keep it. If, on the other hand, it is cool in the spot where you have your culture working,

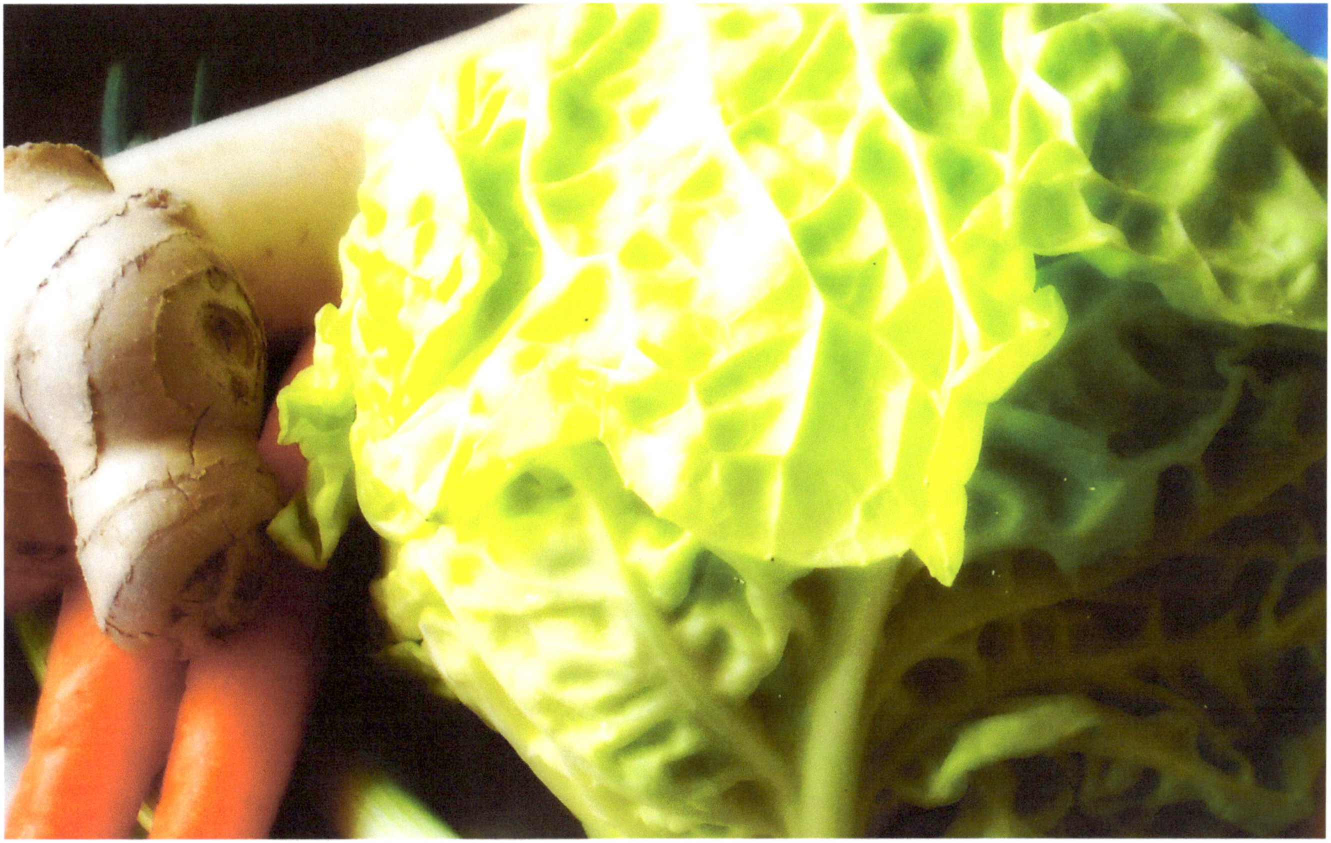

Cranberry Citrus Ferment

Cabbage, chopped, about 70%

Oranges, chopped with skin on, about 10 – 15%

Grapefruit, chopped in very small pieces with skin on, about 5% (optional)

Apples, Granny Smith or Braeburn, about 10 – 15%

Cranberries, fresh or dried, about 5%

Process this recipe the same way as the other two cabbage recipes. Add about a teaspoon of salt for a quart, or 2 teaspoons if you do not have an inoculant. You can use a couple of tablespoons of whey or brine from a previous batch as a culture for a quart. Adjust amounts of different fruits to suit your tastes. This is a unique and wonderful recipe. At our house, we love to put a few tablespoons of the finished product on a bowl of warm oatmeal or warm left-over brown rice with cream or almond milk. Add a sprinkle of cinnamon, a little maple syrup and a few walnuts – delicious!

In a very different setting, this one is good with a mild, white fish or chicken, as well. Also makes a fine topping for a green salad.

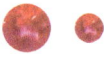

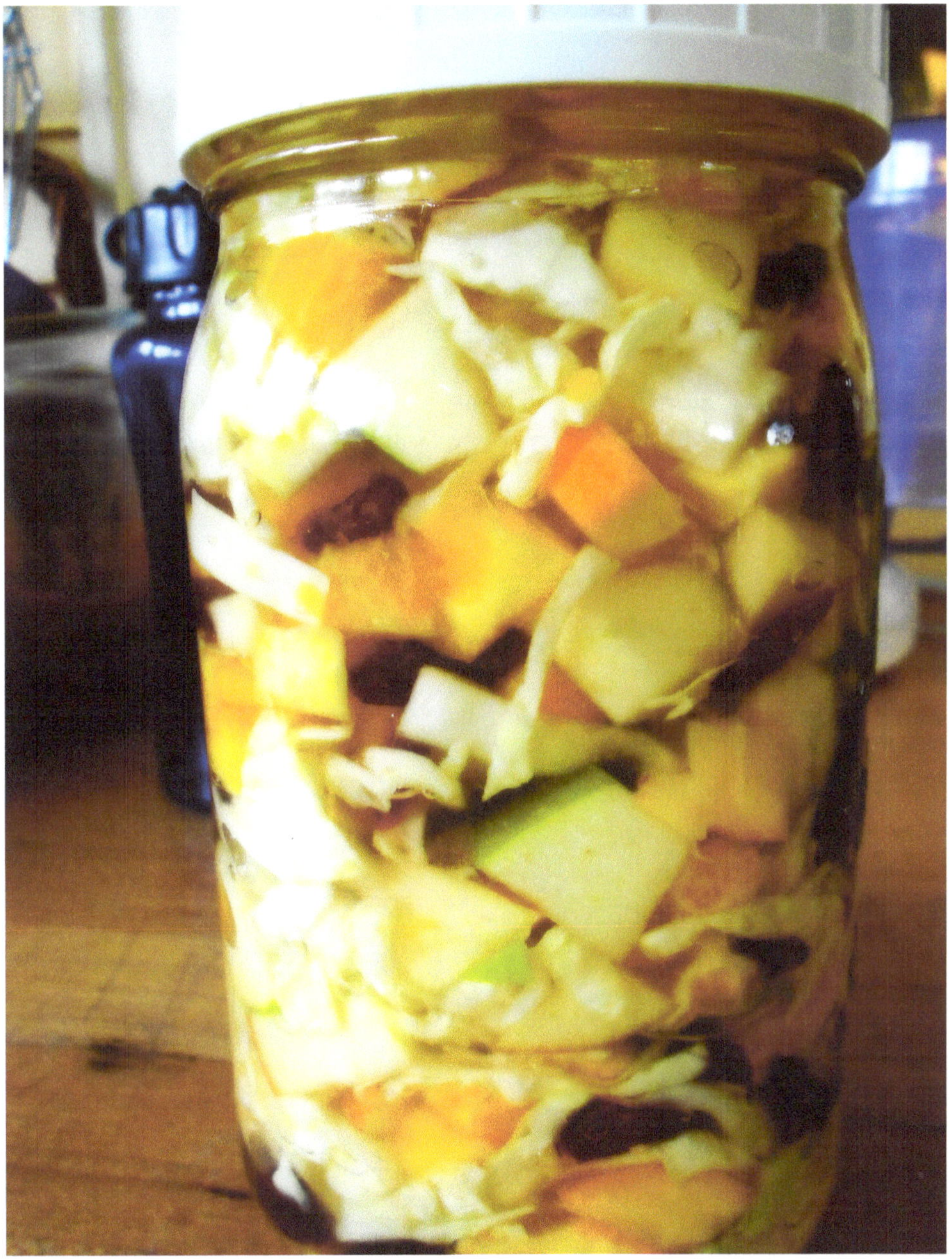

Warming Winter Beets

Red beets, gold beets, or a combination, diced, about 75% of the volume of your container

Carrots, diced, most of the rest of the volume

Ginger root, finely shredded, to taste – about a teaspoon

Minced or finely orange peel, 1-2 tablespoons

Cinnamon, ground, to taste – about ½ teaspoon

I like to use either whey or brine from a previous batch to inoculate this recipe. It's a favorite around our house. It's fabulous as a garnish for many soups and sauces. It goes well with eggs or beef. And, even though the word "winter" appears in the title, the brine makes a very refreshing drink in the summer. I will come in from the garden on a hot day and drink about ½ cup of the stuff, which is also known as "kvass." In researching kvass, I learned that its origins may be Slavic or Russian. It's famous for its cleansing effect on blood and liver, and is prized for its trace minerals and vitamins, including folic acid.

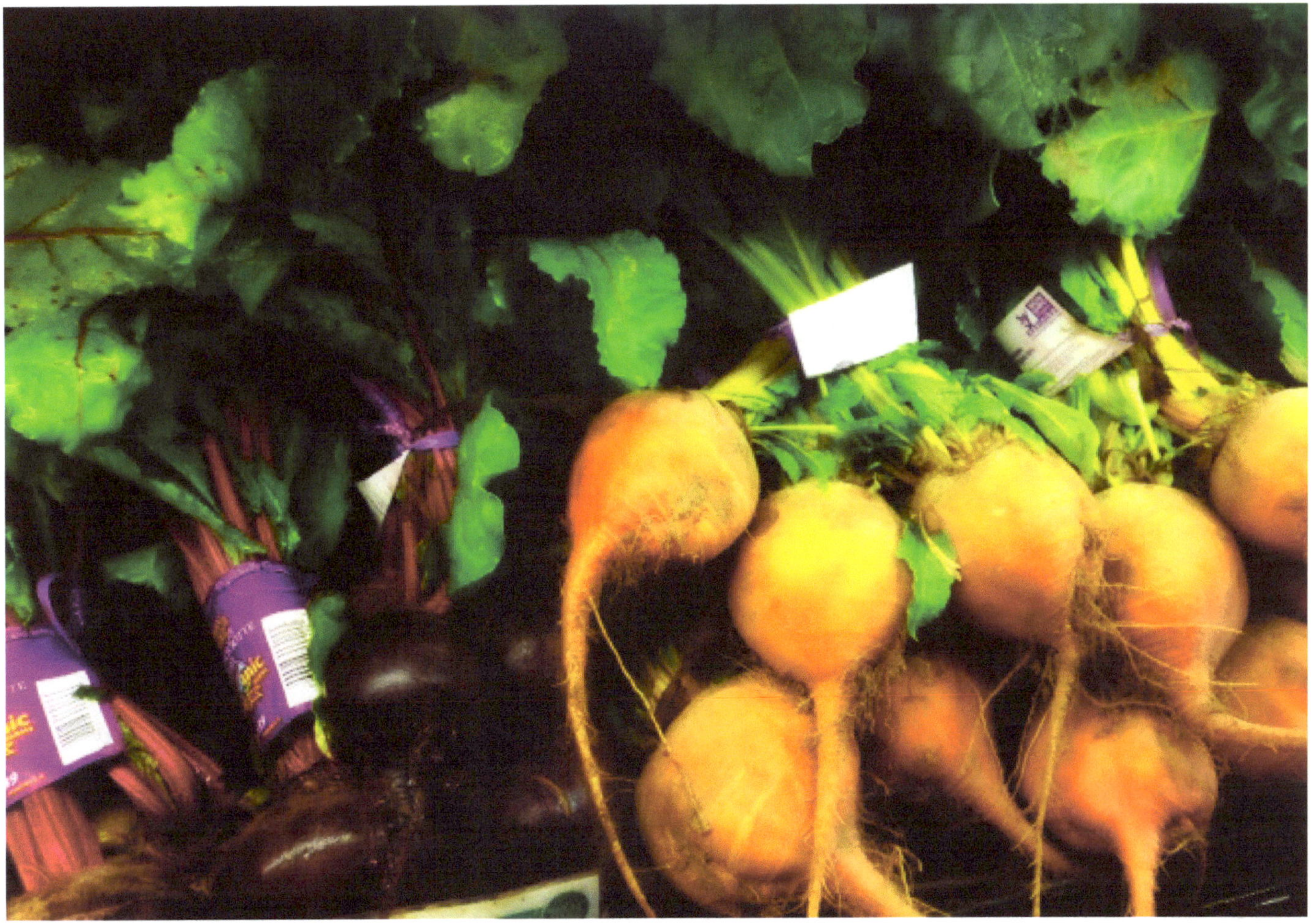

Zucchini and Onions

Zucchini, young and smaller than end-of-summer squash, sliced

Yellow summer squash, sliced

White onion, chopped

I am told that if one includes too many onions or other items from this family (such as garlic), they will not ferment well. I keep the amount of onion in this recipe to about 15 or 20 percent, and I have never had a problem. It's a super-simple recipe, I know! But, again, the smell is sometimes a turn-off. This recipe goes well with Mexican food, and also those sweet bean salads you find in the summer. I'm pretty particular about the hot dogs I eat – no chemical additives and beef only is what I buy- but this ferment is great on a hot dog. Yep, it's a consummate summer dish, for sure.

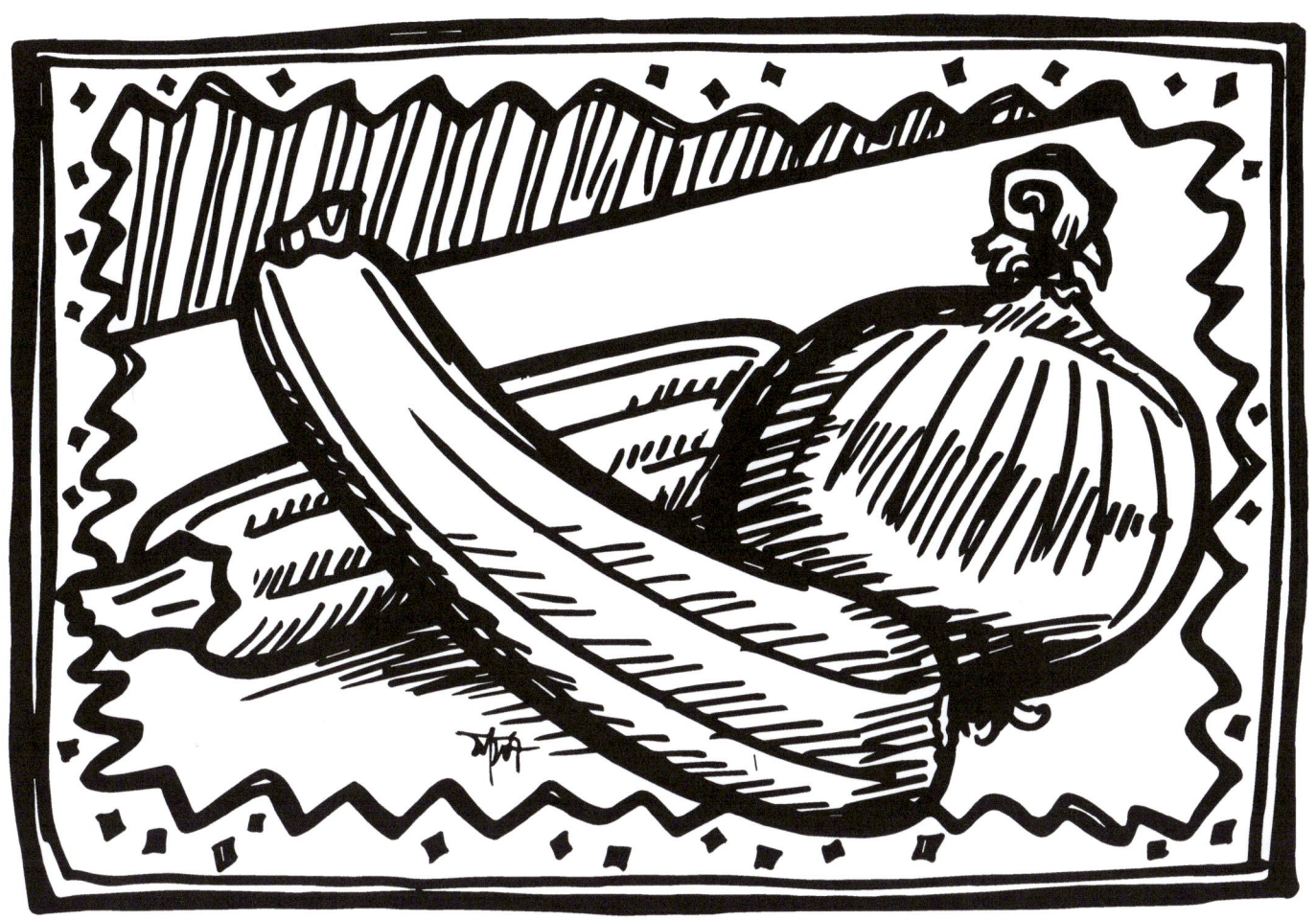

Italian-Stlye Tomatoes

Red tomatoes, chopped, about 40% (These can be canned organic tomatoes or fresh)

Green tomatoes (tomatillos), chopped, about 30%

Green onions, chopped

Black olives, sliced

Fresh basil leaves, chopped

Garlic, fresh & chopped, minced from a jar or garlic powder

Fennel, ground

Black pepper, ground

This recipe is my new personal favorite! I love taking the lid off every day just to smell it. I culture the tomato mixture using whey. It is ready fairly quickly, usually in less than a week. It is fabulous with the squash recipe I will give you next.

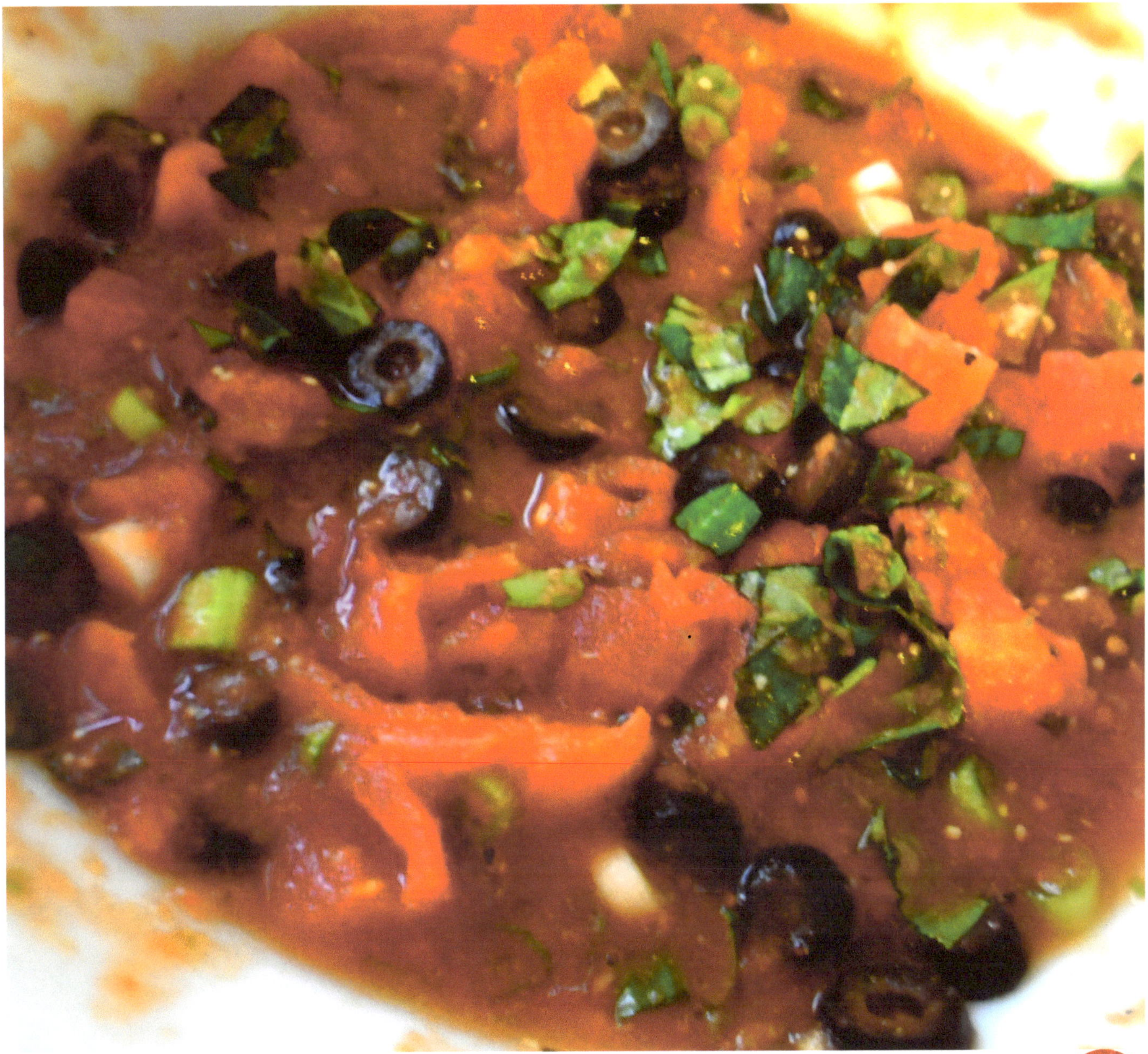

Autumn Spaghetti Squash

Rinse a ripe spaghetti squash and place it in the oven, right on the center rack. Turn oven on to 350 degrees. Let squash bake until it can be pushed in with a firm push of your finger (use a pot holder!) If you want to save the seeds from the squash, you can cut it before baking. Cut vertically and scoop out the seeds and slimy strings from the center of the squash. Place cut-side down in a glass baking dish. Add about 2 cups of water to keep the squash from drying out. Bake for about 25 – 35 minutes.

Once your squash is out of the oven and has cooled sufficiently for you to handle it a bit, you can remove the seeds and inner string/slime, if you have not already done so. Now, with a fork, scrape out the "spaghetti" by lifting the strands away from the skin until only a thin skin is left. Add butter and garlic powder or roasted garlic, and a bit of salt, as you like. I love to also prepare about an equal amount of thin Asian rice noodles to mix with the squash. They are very simple to prepare. Just boil some water, turn heat off and place the noodles in the hot water. Cover and let stand for about 15 minutes while you fix the rest of you meal. Drain off excess water & serve. To the squash and noodles I will usually add a little pasta sauce and the cultured tomatoes. A sprinkle of parmesan cheese is also delicious, if you are a cheese eater.

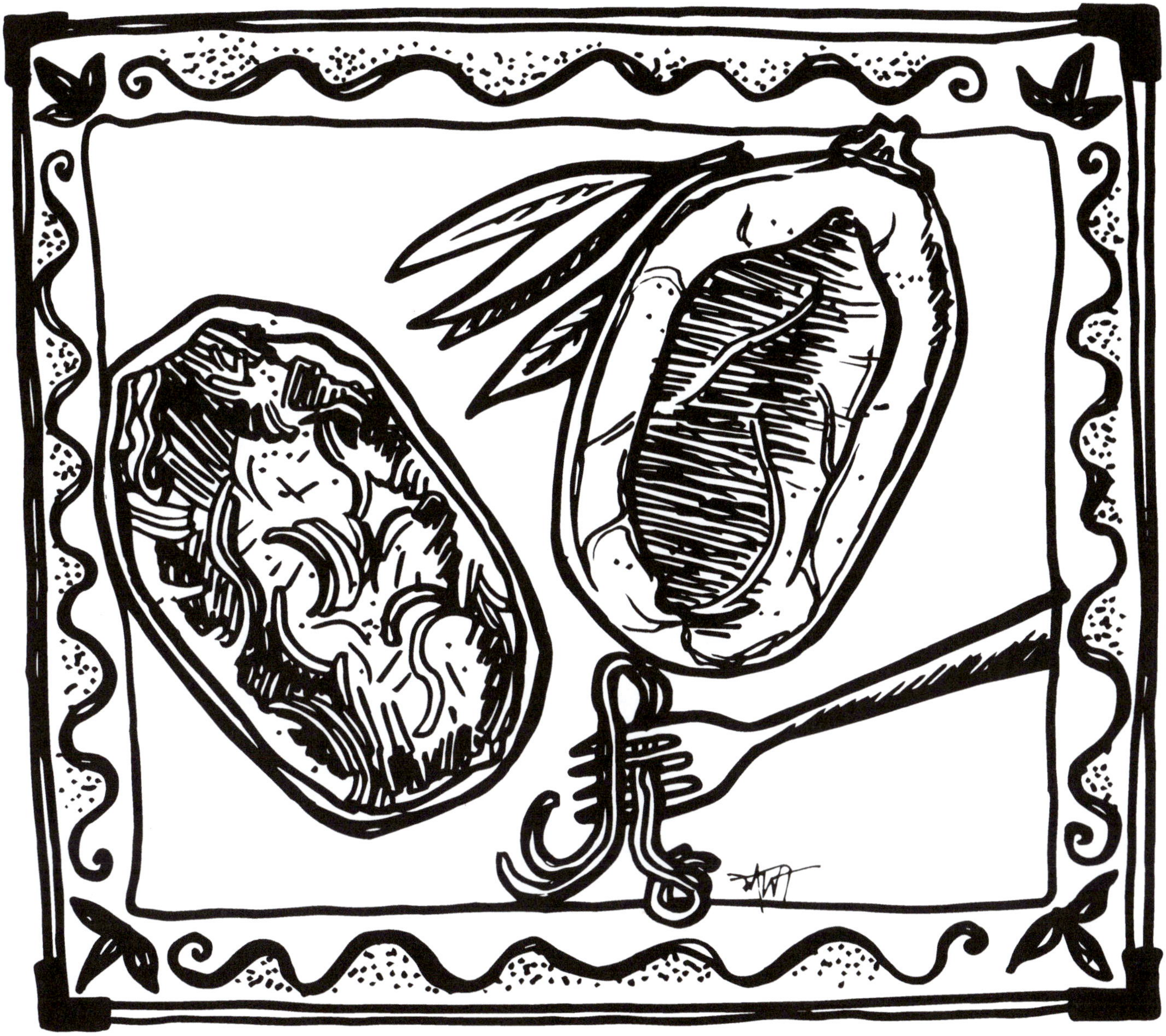

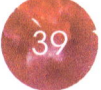

Cultured Fruit Recipes

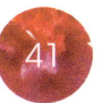

Berries & Pears

2 cups berries, fresh or thawed from frozen, large ones chopped

1 – 2 fresh pears, chopped in pieces similar to size of berries

2 tsp raw honey or maple syrup

Salt, brine from previous batch or whey

    Because fruit ferments so quickly, you can make a nice version of it by simply putting it together the night before you want to use it. Around 24 hours is usually ideal for 69 – 70 degrees, but a little less time is fine. Perfect on pancakes! Just gently stir the fruit together with the honey or syrup and salt, push into the jar firmly enough to release some juice without totally destroying the chunks, add about 1 tablespoon whey or brine, and top with a bit of water if needed. Seal tightly with a lid.

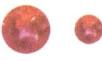

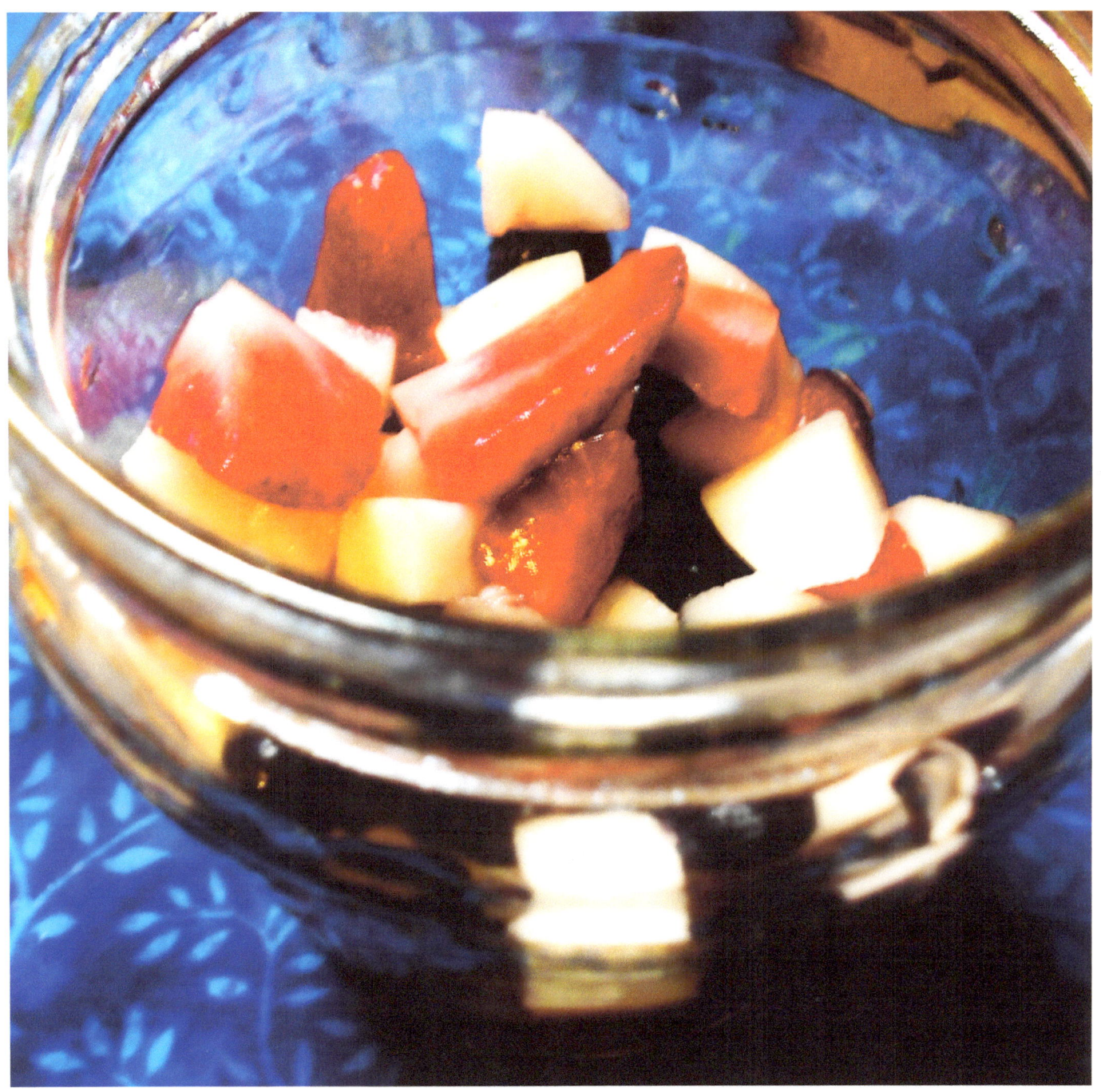

Lemons with Goji

Meyer lemons

Cinnamon sticks

Ground cinnamon

Goji berries

Salt, brine from a previous batch or whey

Cut lemons into quarters, using vertical cuts. If desired, quarters can then be halved. Sprinkle with salt. Press cut lemons into jar, releasing some juice as you press. Sprinkle with a bit of cinnamon as you go. Place cinnamon sticks and goji berries into the jar at intervals. I like to use 1-2 cinnamon sticks, and about 3 tablespoons of goji berries for a quart jar, but vary the amounts to suit your tastes.

For some reason, these lemons always want to sneak up above the line of liquid in the jar, no matter what I try! The best thing seems to be to make sure they are covered with lemon juice, adding water if needed to the top, and seal the jar up tightly (being careful, once again, to leave about an inch of space at the top of the jar for expansion). I check the jar nearly every day by inspecting it without opening, and every few days by opening and poking the lemons down again. I usually let these ferment for about a month.

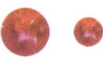

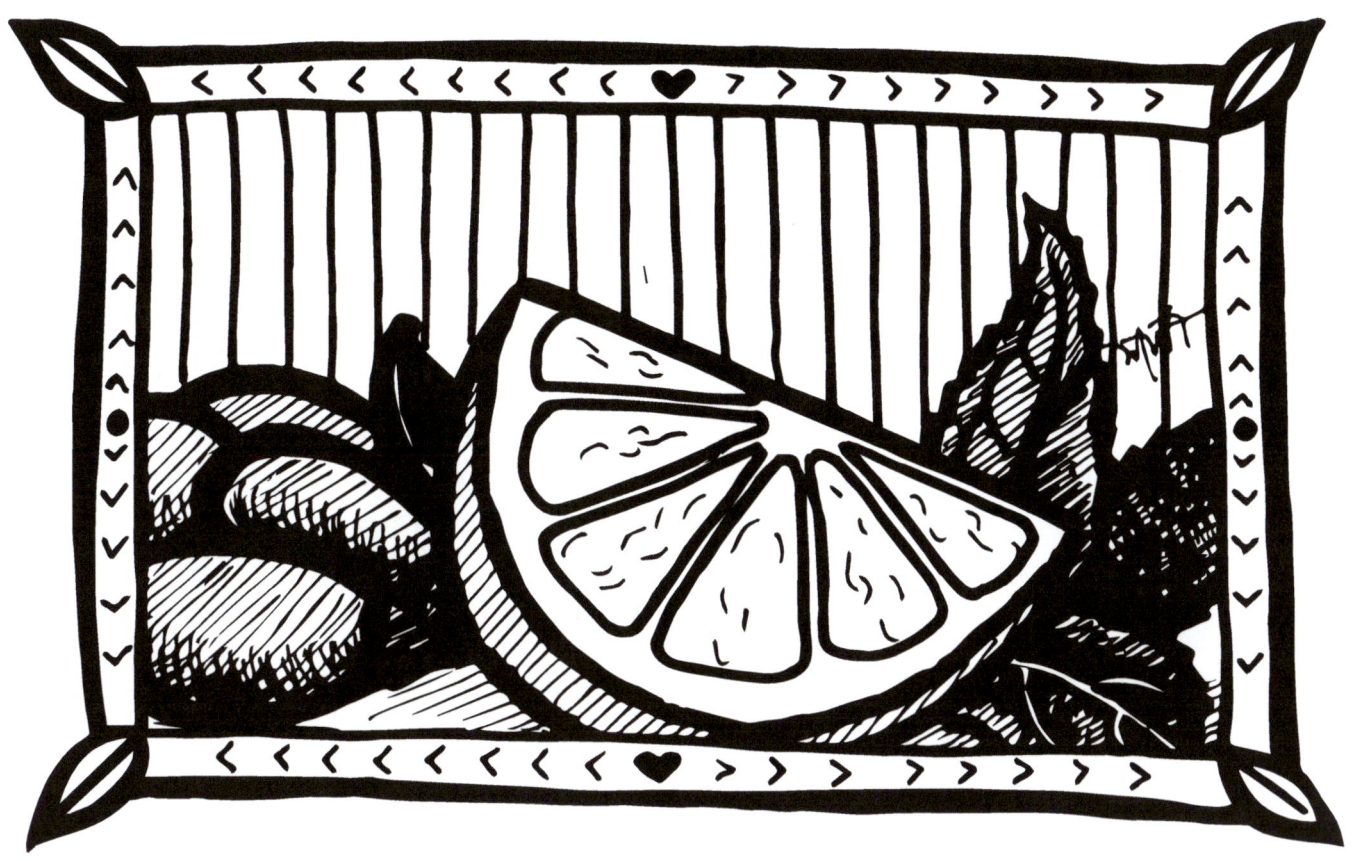

Cultured lemons are usually called "preserved lemons," and are known for bringing their unique flavor (especially when paired with olives) to Moroccan dishes such as chicken tagines. They can also be wonderful with gluten free pasta salads and baked goods. The best results can be had when using Meyer lemons, due to their sweeter flavor and thin rind. However, if you can't find Meyers, you can use regular lemons. If the rind is very thick, you may want to remove some or most of it. I really enjoy the way the rind ferments, but too much of it is, well, too much!

Mango Peach Ferment

This little recipe has a kick to it that will liven up breakfast! Enjoy it with eggs or gluten free waffles or pancakes. It's also a fine addition to fish, tacos, or Indian food. Mangoes are a bit tricky if you're not accustomed to choosing fresh ones. The ones at the peak of ripeness look to me as if they are already going bad – dingy color, wrinkled skin- but that's how to find the best ones. The bright, smooth ones are usually hard as a rock, difficult to slice and taste awful. You could use frozen mangoes for this recipe. Just thaw them first. Of course, you could also use frozen berries and peaches, but the best way to do this is to prepare this culture with fresh peaches when they are in season.

> Mangoes, diced
>
> Peaches, diced (about equal amount to mangoes)
>
> Blueberries (about ¼ as much as other fruits)
>
> Turmeric (1/2 teaspoon for a quart)
>
> Fennel seeds, slightly hammered
>
> Mustard seeds, slightly hammered
>
> Hot sauce, to taste
>
> Celery juice, fresh
>
> (if you don't have a juicer, either borrow one or just use water)

Small amount of salt, whey, or brine from a previous batch If using brine or whey, use about a tablespoon for a quart jar. In this case, I would leave out the additional salt, due to the sodium in the celery juice. A very light sprinkle of salt is all that is needed, even without whey or brine. If you use water instead of celery juice, use a similar amount of salt to the other fruit recipes, about ½ teaspoon for a quart (or more if you do not inoculate).

Gently toss ingredients in a bowl, except for juice. Place into jar and gently press down with wooden spoon. Add a small amount of celery juice until fruit is completely covered. Close jar with a tight-fitting lid and let the mixture culture at room temperature. It will not take long – as little as 8 hours will do the trick. If your room is cooler, you may let it ferment for up to 24 hours. Place finished ferment in the fridge where it can be safely stored for about a month.

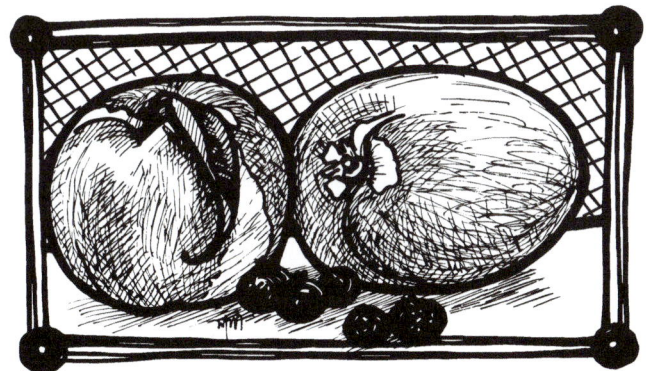

Beverages

Kombucha

By now, you've probably noticed bottles of this phenomenal beverage in your local grocery store. It's becoming quite popular, and yet, usually when I share this drink with a client or friend for the first time, the response is something between, "That's really weird," and, "That's disgusting! How can you stand to drink this stuff?" I think it's a bit of an acquired taste, because these same people often show up later with a bottle of the stuff in hand, hooked like the rest of us!

According to Tom Valentine, author of Search For Health, kombucha tea is a powerful detoxifier, due to a substance called glucuronic acid. Glucuronic acid is produced by humans in the liver, and "binds up" toxins and poisons from any source, escorting them from the body via the excretory system. These toxic substances, once bound, cannot be resorbed by the body. So, the SCOBY (which we'll discuss in a moment) feeds on the sugar & tea, then produces acetic, lactic and glucuronic acids – all beneficial to us.

Kombucha tea is remarkably easy to brew at home and not expensive at all. You may not realize this if you've been buying the commercially available ones. The bottled kombucha in the stores is wonderful stuff; don't get me wrong. But it costs a bit more than a soda, or most any other single serving beverage in the refrigerator. To brew it at home, you only need a few things and a little time.

Let's begin with the tea. There is a type of tea called "jun" that is made

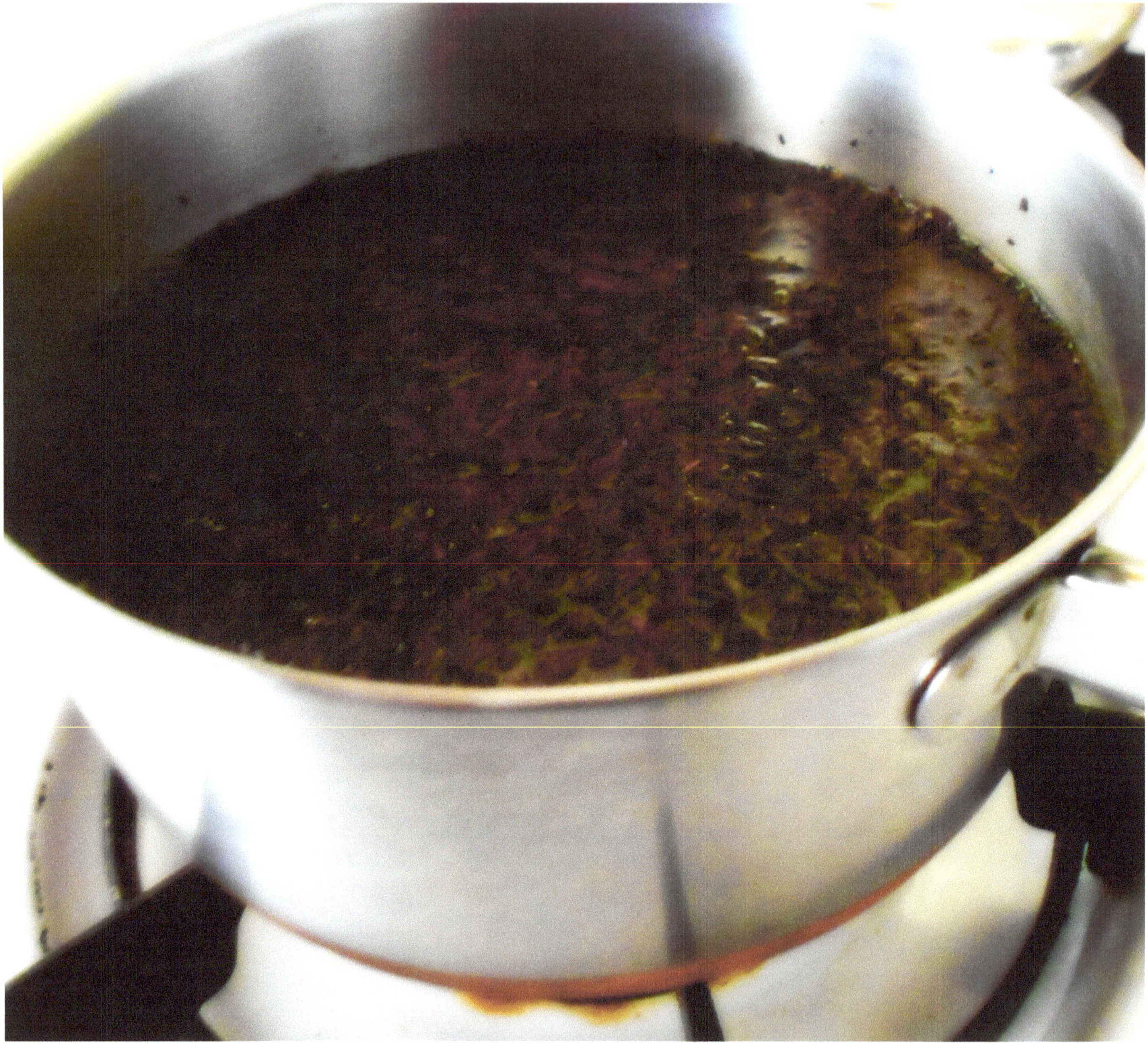

using green tea. For kombucha, you'll want to start with black tea. I like to use a nice loose-leaf tea, because I don't care to have paper in my compost pile that I did not really need in the first place. However, if you use tea bags, you'll want to start with about 3 for a half gallon jar. For loose tea, use about 3-4 teaspoons.

This leads me to the next thing you'll need: a jar. Of course, you can use a gallon jar, or a larger one. What I recommend to clients, and what I do myself, is to drink only about 4 to 8 ounces per day of kombucha. I do not even drink it every day, but several times per week. Some people can have adverse reactions to

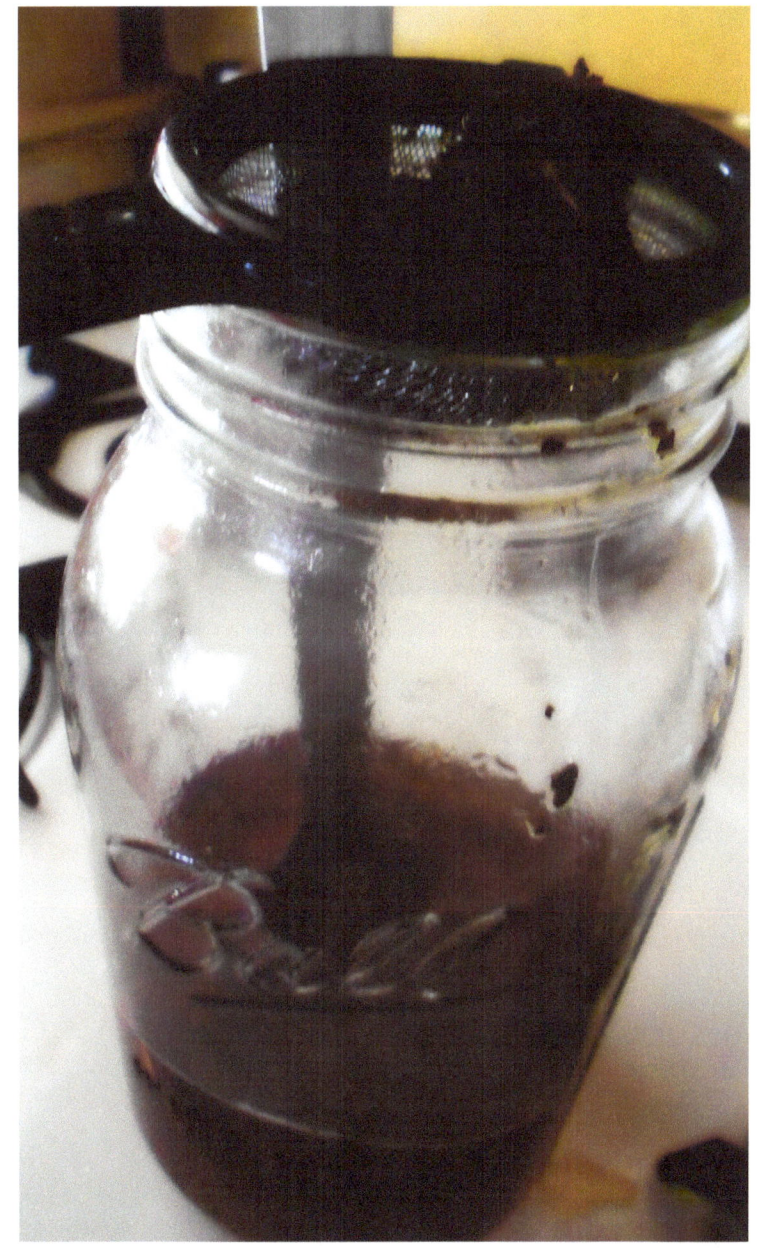

large amounts of kombucha. It also does have sugar in it. You may read about how the SCOBY consumes the sugar, and that is true – sort of. I really don't fully understand the science, and why this point is debated at all, but it seems that some sugar remains in the final product, and as such, you may want to limit your consumption of it. What I'm trying to say is simply that I use a half gallon jar for the tea, as opposed to a larger one, because that is enough for me. 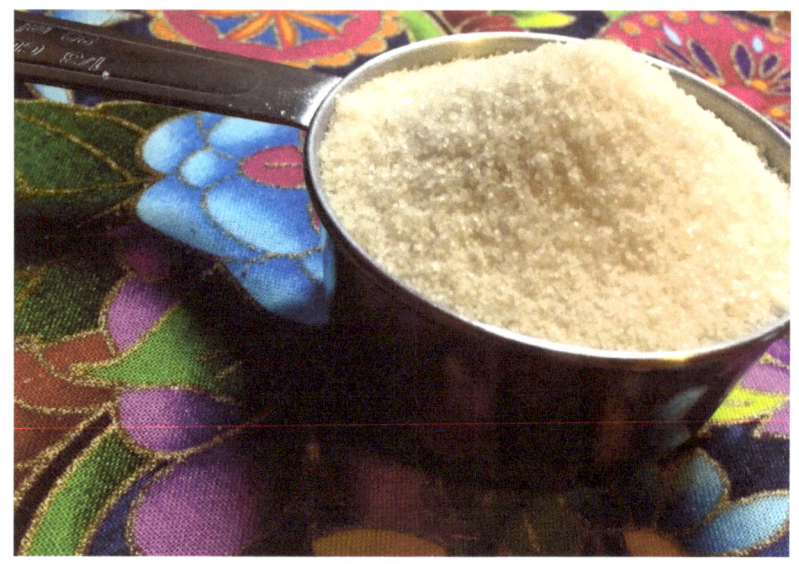 Perhaps you noticed the next thing you will need to make kombucha: sugar. I use organic sugar, but beyond that, there's nothing special about it. I have read that the sugar is absolutely essential, and I have tried making the kombucha using fruit juice instead of sugar, so I could avoid using the "evil" stuff. However, my experiment failed, so I just use sugar. For a half gallon, I put in a bit more than 1/3 cup.

The critical ingredient for making kombucha is a SCOBY, which stands for

"symbiotic culture of bacteria and yeast." It is sometimes called a "kombucha mushroom," and looks fairly creepy as it hangs in the
tea. As your tea brews, a "baby" will grow underneath the "mother" SCOBY that you begin with. You can
acquire a SCOBY by searching online – it's easy, I promise! You can often find one by chatting to locals in your natural grocery store; since the SCOBY naturally multiplies, people enjoy giving them away.

If you purchase kombucha tea, you can sort of cheat by using most of a bottle of this tea instead of a full SCOBY. Try to choose a bottle that has some visible floating "gunk." Add it to your tea at the appropriate time, careful not to pour it in when the tea is hot, as we will discuss below.

You will want something in which to brew your tea. I use a stainless steel sauce pan with a lid, and a strainer to remove the tea leaves. Bring about 2 – 3 cups of water (many experts recommend using filtered, and that would be great) to nearly boiling. Add tea leaves or bags to water and cover with lid. Brew for desired length of time (I steep for about 2 minutes; long brew times make bitter tea.)

Next, you can prepare your jar. Use a clean jar. For this recipe (1/2 gallon), you will first add about a cup of cool water to the jar. Now, place a long-handled stainless steel spoon or other utensil in the jar. These steps will prevent the jar breaking from the heat of the tea. Place the strainer over the top of the jar, and slowly pour the tea into the jar with the water, straining out the tea leaves.

Now you are ready to add the sugar. Your tea is still warm, so the sugar will dissolve easily as you gently stir the sugar into the tea. Once sugar is fully dissolved, add cold water to within about 3 – 4 inches of the top of the jar. Test the temperature of the tea by placing your hands on the jar for a few seconds. It should be just barely warm to touch. If it feels very warm, let it cool for a half hour and come back. Too much heat would kill your SCOBY!

This is the time you can add your starter kombucha tea to the batch. I use 1/3 cup. (If you do not have a SCOBY, you can brew this tea using a full bottle, or most of a bottle, of kombucha from the store.) Then, using a wooden spoon, transfer your SCOBY gently to the top of the jar. It will probably float on the top, but if it slips in sideways and hangs midway in the tea, that's okay.
I have seen variations in brewing time for kombucha ranging from a week to a month. Give it a taste to see if it is ready after a week or so, depending on the temperature of your environment. The taste should be a bit sour, but not too vinegary. It may be a bit fizzy (lucky you!) If you want to try differing lengths of time for fermentation, dip some of the kombucha out and put it in a jar in the refrigerator. Let the rest continue to brew, tasting every couple of days until you

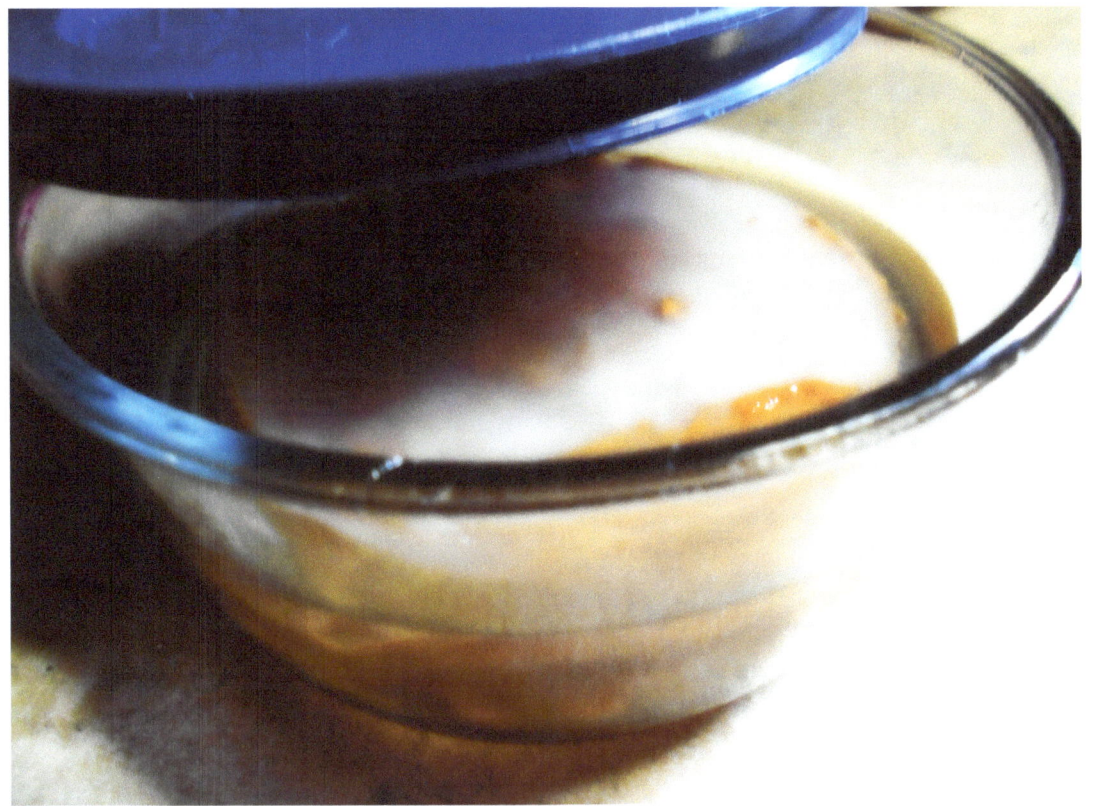

are satisfied. Now you can compare this to your first harvest from your fridge
.

    Something I sometimes do in the summer is to brew a large jar of kombucha, as described above, and dip out enough to fill a bottle to place in the fridge. I brew a cup or 2 of fresh tea, stir in a little sugar, let it cool, then add it to the big jar and let it ferment for a few days. Then, I do the same every few days. In this way, I have a continuous brew. If I want to drink more, I just replace whatever I dip out with fresh black tea.

Flavors

What about all the wonderful flavors you can find at the store? The best way I have found to flavor my kombucha is the method I will share with you now. When the kombucha is ready to be bottled, I take a few bottles and place in each one about ¾ cup of fruit juice or a mixture of juices. I sometimes use a juice made with fresh ginger, which can be quite strong by itself, but is glorious in the kombucha.

Once the juice is in the bottles, I fill each one with kombucha and screw the lids on tightly. There are some terrific bottles available online, but I just reuse the ones from the store. I then place the bottles on the counter to ferment for about 1 - 3 more days. The juice ferments, and the whole concoction is delicious!

If, by mistake, you over-ferment your kombucha and it tastes too vinegary, do not despair! Use it as vinegar! It makes some wonderful salad dressings and can be reduced for a lovely sauce.

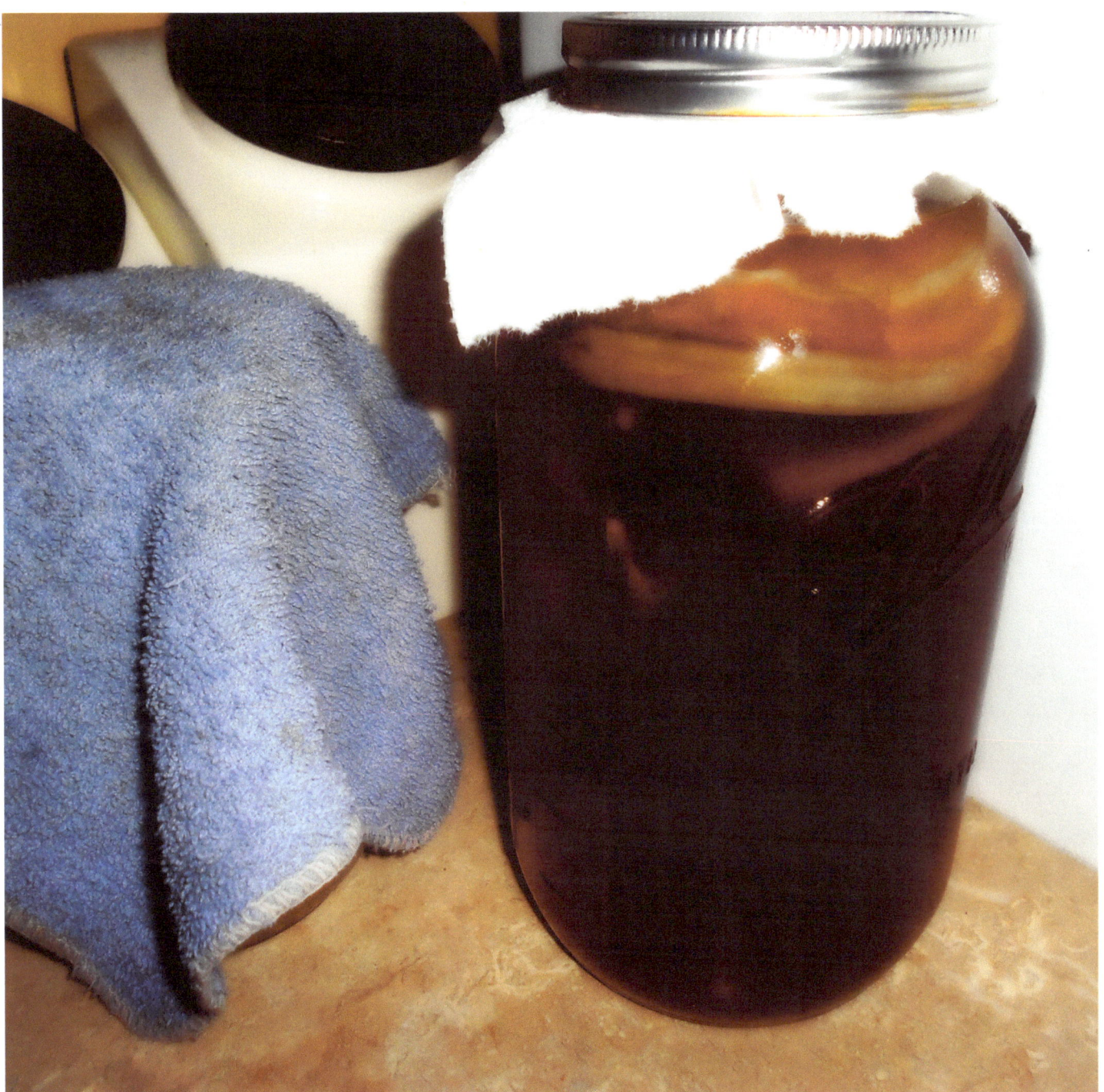

Green Veggie Juice With Green Tea

If you have a juicer at home, you will be able to put this delicious drink together quickly. It takes a short ferment time, so you'll be able to enjoy drinking it tomorrow!

Begin with 1 quart of freshly brewed green tea. When I researched the brewing of green teas, there was a vast amount of information about varieties, harvest times, the age of your tea (should not have been on your kitchen shelf for the last 5 years), temperatures of water for brewing and length of brewing time. The water you use can affect your final product, too, of course.

Generally, I recommend you use water that has not come to the boiling point, but close, and is around 160 degrees. For a quart of green tea, I like to use about a tablespoon of tea leaves, or 3 to 4 teabags. I will brew it for about 2 minutes, or slightly less. For this recipe, I brew the tea, strain out the tea leaves, cover and let it cool while I make the juice.

For the juice, you will want to select fresh veggies and cut them to the size and shape required by your juicer.

Celery, 3 -5 long stalks, depending upon size

Cucumber, 1 small or ½ large

Spinach, 1 cup

Carrot, 1

Granny smith apple, ½

Whey for culture, 1 teaspoon

Adjust amounts of ingredients to your own tastes. Combine juice and warm tea in a large pitcher or jar. Be sure overall temperature of this mixture is not too warm. It should feel just lukewarm to the touch. Heat kills culture, so you want to check this before adding the whey. When whey is added to the jar, cover with a lid or towel. Place out of direct sunlight in a place that will stay around 70 degrees for about 24 hours. If temperature is 72-75 degrees, check after 8 – 12 hours. Too long will produce a vinegary drink.

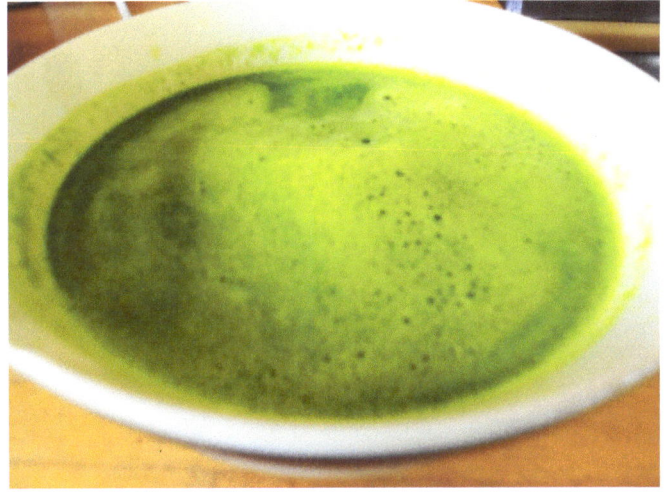

Ginger Ale

Ginger ale was a favorite of mine as a child, but it was never like this! This refreshing fermented ale is more than sugar and bubbles. Using fresh ginger and citrus juice makes it flavorful and culturing it loads it up with salubrious, easy to absorb electrolytes. See how long a jar lasts in your refrigerator!

- 1 ½ cups fresh grated ginger root
- ½ cup fresh squeezed lime juice
- ½ cup fresh squeezed lemon juice
- ¾ cup organic sugar or ½ cup raw unfiltered honey
- 1 tablespoon salt
- ½ cup whey
- **Water to fill half gallon jar**

When preparing ginger, the easiest way I have found to grate it is to first freeze it, then grate it using a fine grater. Start with adding your ginger to the jar, add the rest of the ingredients, straining out any
lemon seeds. If your water is about room temperature or slightly warmer, the honey will mix in well (if you use honey). Stir it all up, put the lid on and let it sit on a counter, out of direct sunlight for 2 to 3 days. Transfer to the refrigerator. Server by straining out grated ginger and mixing half and half with mineral water. But don't throw the ginger away! Use it in a batch of muffins or toss it into a salad dressing.

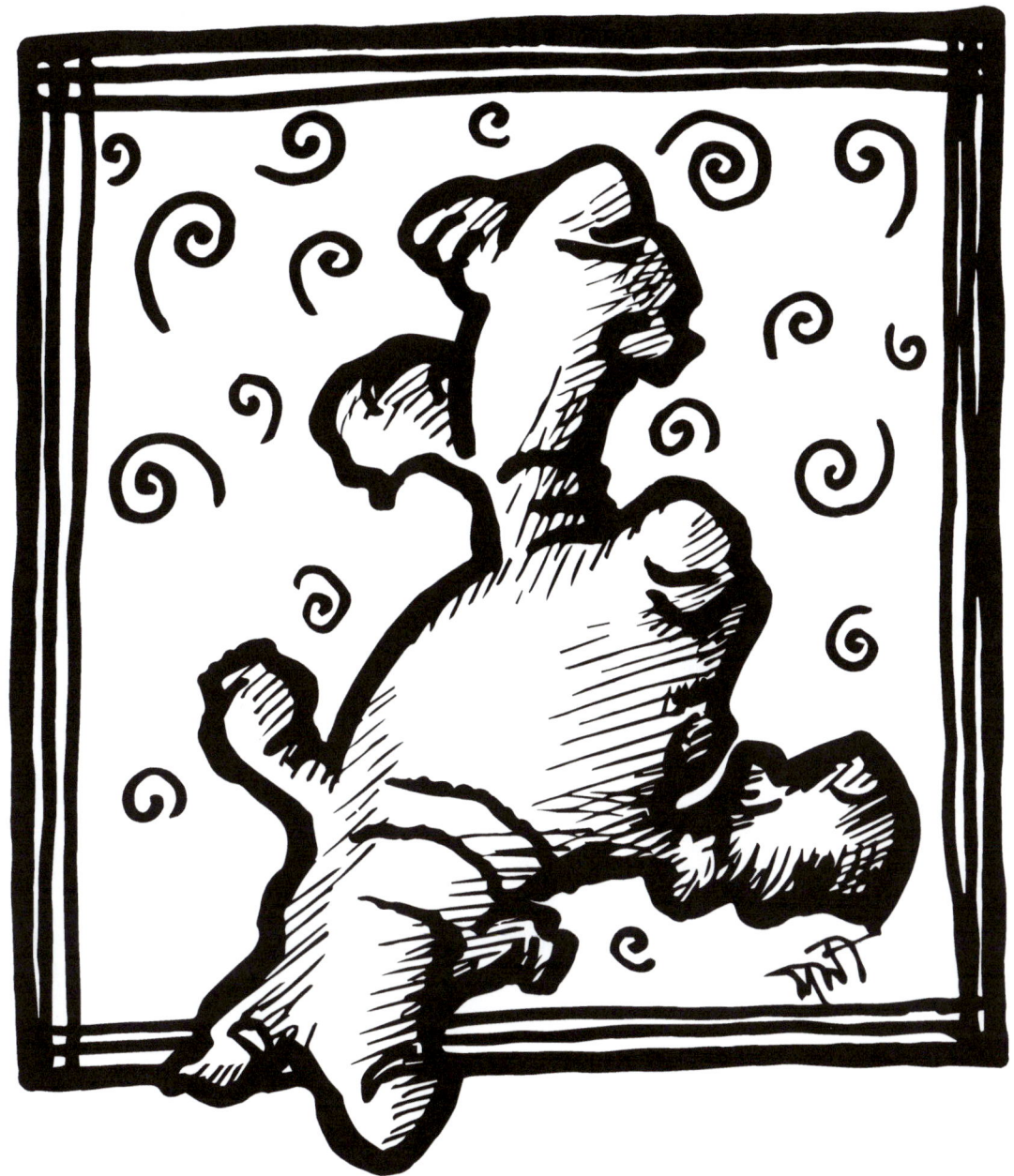

Condiments

Culturing your condiments is so easy! It's also an easy way to have a fermented food with every meal, since they usually stay in the fridge for weeks. Even when my family decides to grill burgers or all beef, uncured organic hot dogs, I can spread some cultured mustard on my gluten free bun, and maybe a little sauerkraut, too. Delicious!

Easy Cultured Mustard

½ cup pickle brine from cultured pickles, if available (otherwise, use water)

1 tablespoon whey

1 tablespoon finely minced onion

1 tablespoon finely minced garlic

½ cup mustard seeds – I like to use about a 4 to 1 ration of yellow to brown, but use more brown seeds for a spicier mustard, or use all mustard for mild.

½ teaspoon salt, if no brine is available

1 teaspoon pure maple syrup

Combine all ingredients except salt & syrup in a bowl. Soak for 8-12 hours at room temperature. Then, blend or process, adding maple syrup and salt (if used). May take a few minutes to become smooth. Store in a glass jar with a lid in the refrigerator for up to several months.

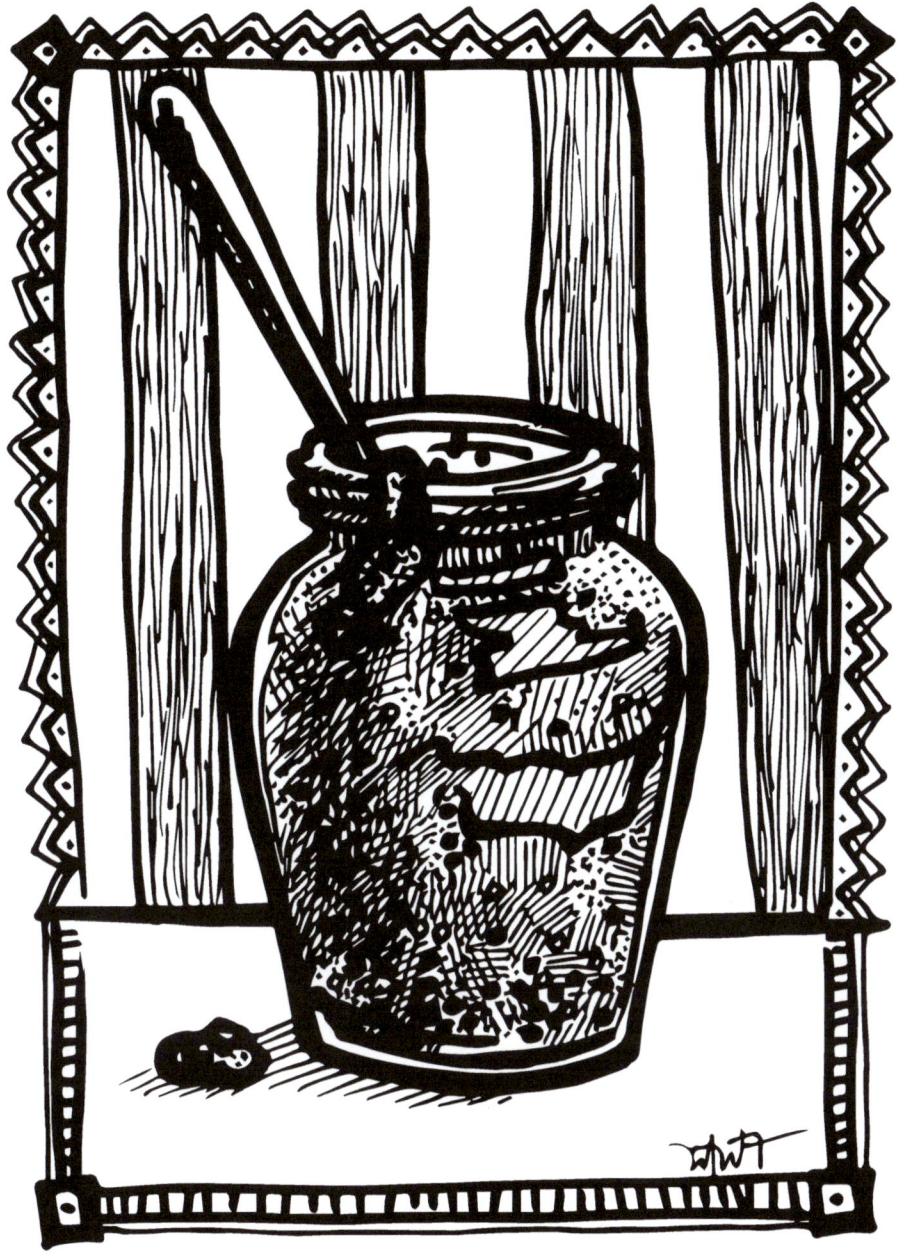

Mango Salsa

For this salsa, I use a prepared chipotle sauce, or a bit of canned chipotle pepper. I love the smoky flavor, but these peppers are almost too hot for me. Using the prepared sauce makes it easy to use just the right amount. Feel free to add more if you can take the heat!

- Green tomatillos and red tomatoes, chopped - half of each, to make about 50% of the total volume.
- Mangoes and pineapples, chopped - about half of each, to make about 20% of the total volume
- Cilantro, chopped – use a generous handful
- Minced garlic
- Salt & black pepper
- Whey – ¼ cup for a quart jar

Mix all ingredients in a large bowl. Place into desired jar(s), leaving at least 1 inch of empty space at the top of each jar. Cover tightly. This recipe ferments quickly! The jar I have in my fridge is slightly effervescent, but very tasty. At 70 degrees, this salsa could be ready in as little as 8 to 12 hours.

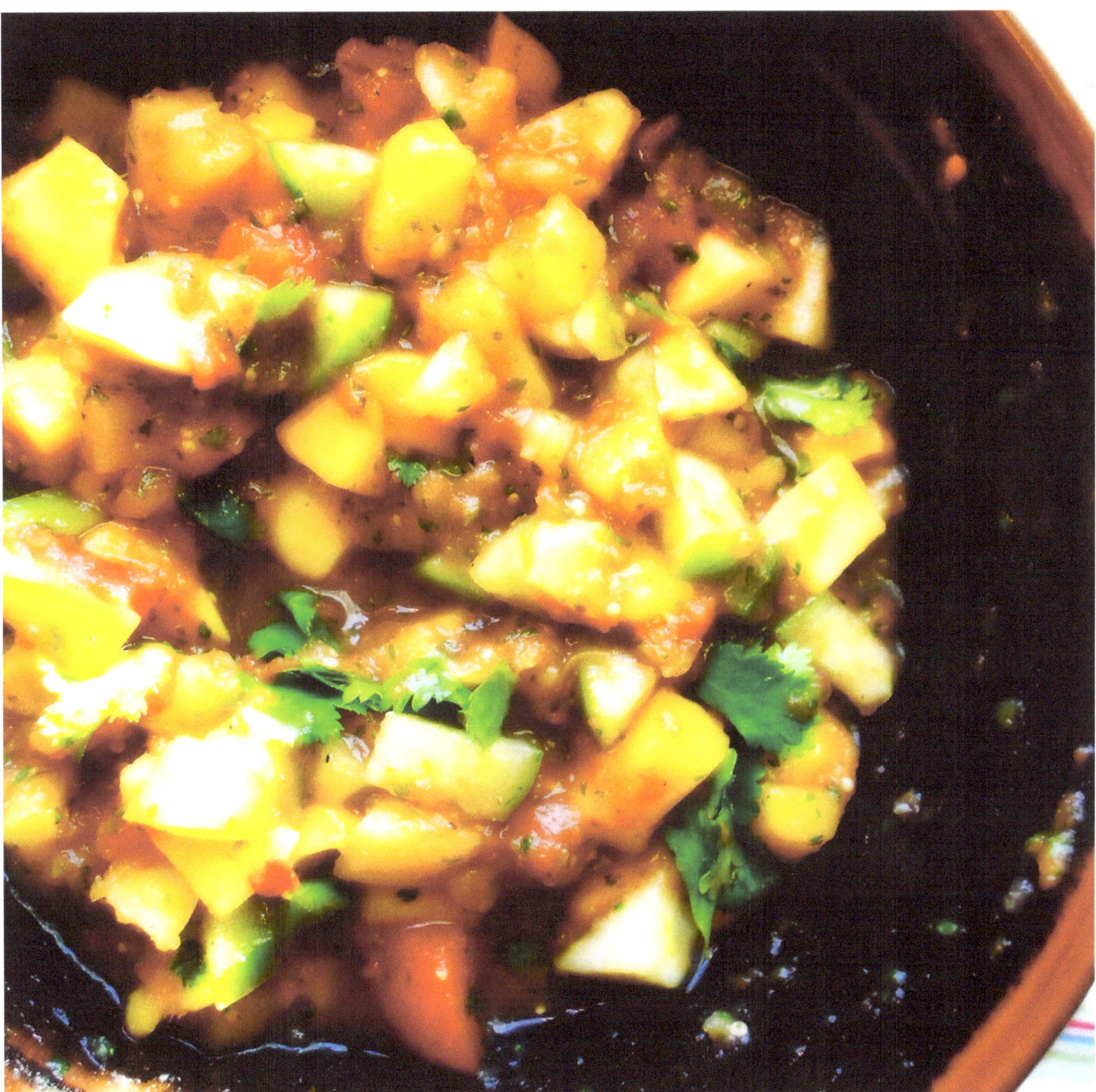

Lacto Fermented Ketchup

You could make this recipe from scratch if you wanted to begin by making your own tomato paste, but I never seem to have enough tomatoes on hand to do that. A good quality commercial one will still yield marvelous ketchup, however.

- 2 cups tomato paste
- 1/8 cup mixture of molasses & maple syrup
- 1/8 cup peach, mango or plum puree
- 3 tablespoons raw apple cider vinegar (or the best quality commercial one you can get)
- 1 teaspoon sea salt
- 1 teaspoon allspice
- ½ teaspoon ground cloves
- ¼ cup plus 2 tablespoons whey, divided

Whisk all ingredients together, except 2 tablespoons whey. Top with remaining whey by spooning gently on top, and loosely cover with a dish towel. Let sit at room temperature for 5 to 7 days to culture. When finished culturing, stir well, put lid on jar and refrigerate for up to several months.

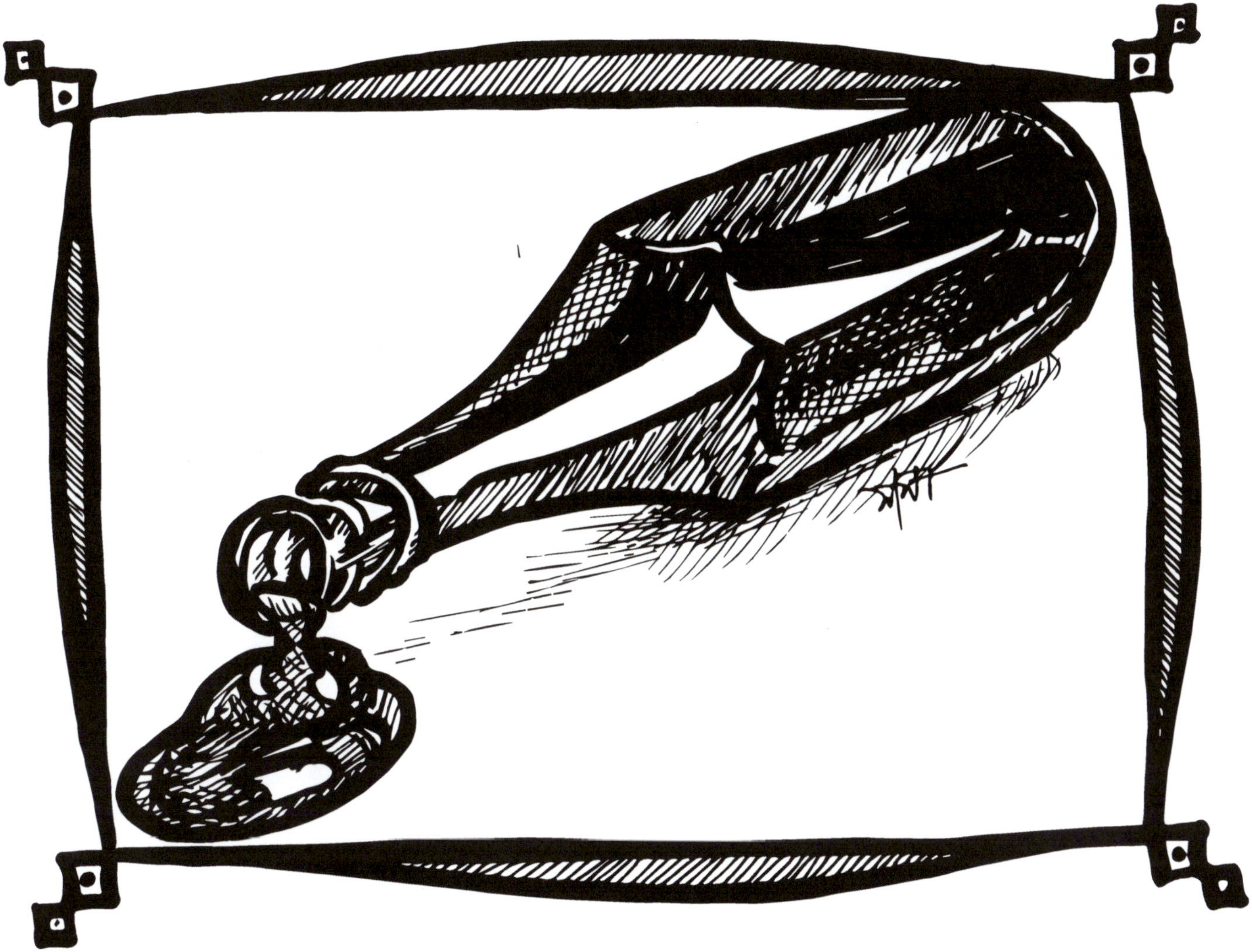

69

Sourdough

These days, lots of folks are having a tough time digesting grains. Some experts believe that this is a result of abandoning some traditional ways of preparing grain. Others maintain that we have made changes to our grains through hybridization, to our detriment. Still others believe that we have simply made grains too great a percentage of our overall diets. In any case, we can counter some of the problems from grains by souring our dough before baking or cooking.

Souring is a traditional technique that helps neutralize anti-nutrients, especially phytic acid. Phytic acid blocks absorption of important minerals, and is present in the outer coatings of nuts and seeds. Additionally, souring grains, like other methods of fermentation, multiplies nutrients, notably the B vitamins, but also others. It also has the effect of lowering the glycemic index. It's easy to do, and takes only a little time and planning. In fact, I think these recipes actually come together more quickly than others. Or, maybe it just feels that way because they only take a few minutes at a time.

Sourdough Pancakes

½ cup buckwheat flour

½ cup brown rice flour

2 tablespoons plain yogurt (this is important – there must be NO added sugar!) If you are sensitive to casein or lactose, you can use whey or liquid acidophilus instead of yogurt.

The night before you want to make the pancakes, mix these 3 ingredients together in a mixing bowl, adding just enough water to make a sort of thick paste. Cover with a lid or plate, and leave it sitting at room temperature overnight. The next morning, you are ready for part 2.

To the bowl add:

1 egg (farm fresh free range, if possible)

2 tablespoons melted butter or coconut oil

½ teaspoon baking soda

¼ teaspoon salt

I like to mix this up with a fork. You could also use a whisk, especially if you double the recipe. If the batter is too thick, add a little water or coconut milk. Cook on a hot skillet, using butter or coconut oil to keep them from sticking. I use these 2 fats for cooking because, unlike other plant oils, they are chemically stable at reasonable cooking temperatures. When bubbles appear & pancakes appear dry around the edges, flip with a spatula and cook on the other side for about a minute. My family lives these served with almond butter and pure maple syrup. Feel free to try all your favorite toppings!

Yam Muffins

2/3 cup brown rice flour

1/3 cup millet flour

1/3 cup white rice flour

1/3 cup gluten free rolled oats

1 cup water

2 tablespoons plain kefir or yogurt

Stir all the above ingredients together to mix well. Cover and let stand overnight, or between 8 and 24 hours. Now you are ready for part 2.

1 cup shredded yam

½ cup each chopped pistachios and shredded unsweetened coconut

2 tablespoons melted butter

2 eggs

4 tablespoons raw honey

20 pods cardamom, ground

1 teaspoon baking soda

¼ teaspoon salt

Add remaining ingredient to bowl and stir well, or add them first to a Nutri-Bullet and blend for about 20 seconds, then add this mixture to the bowl and stir well. (I like to use this method.) Fill cups of a muffin tin about 2/3 full. Bake at 350 degrees Fahrenheit for about 14 minutes. Let them cool in the pan for a few minutes, then serve warm with butter or cultured fruit

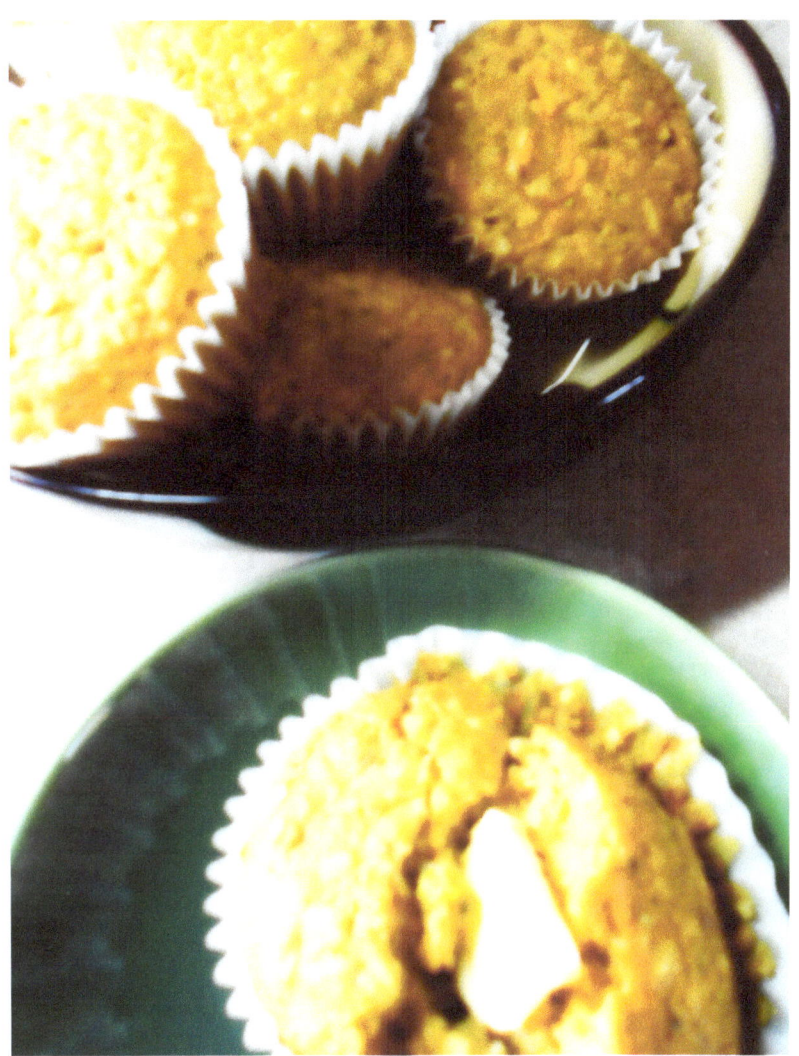

Cultured Oatmeal

This is not technically "sourdough," but it is a delicious soured grain, so here we go. It's so simple to make soured, or cultured oatmeal that I make it regularly in the winter. It's hearty and warm, and keeps me filled up for hours, unlike any instant variety. It takes about the same amount of time in the morning as instant, too!

The night prior to your oatmeal adventure, start with the following ingredients:

1 cup gluten free rolled oats, or steel cut oats

Enough water to just cover oats in a bowl

2 teaspoons miso

Stir minimally, cover and let the oatmeal sit out for 8 to 12 hours at room temperature. The next morning, it will be ready to cook. Figs may also be prepared the night before by placing 5 or 6 mission or Calimyrna figs in a glass jar and covering with 1 cup water and a lid. Place closed jar in the refrigerator overnight.

Bring 1 cup of water to boil in a sauce pan over medium heat. Add cultured oats to boiling water and stir while cooking for about 2 to 3 minutes. Add more water if desired, or add coconut, almond or dairy milk. Remove from heat and add 2 tablespoons almond butter. Cover to keep warm while preparing figs. Remove figs from water, remove any stems and chop figs. Add figs to oatmeal stir and serve.

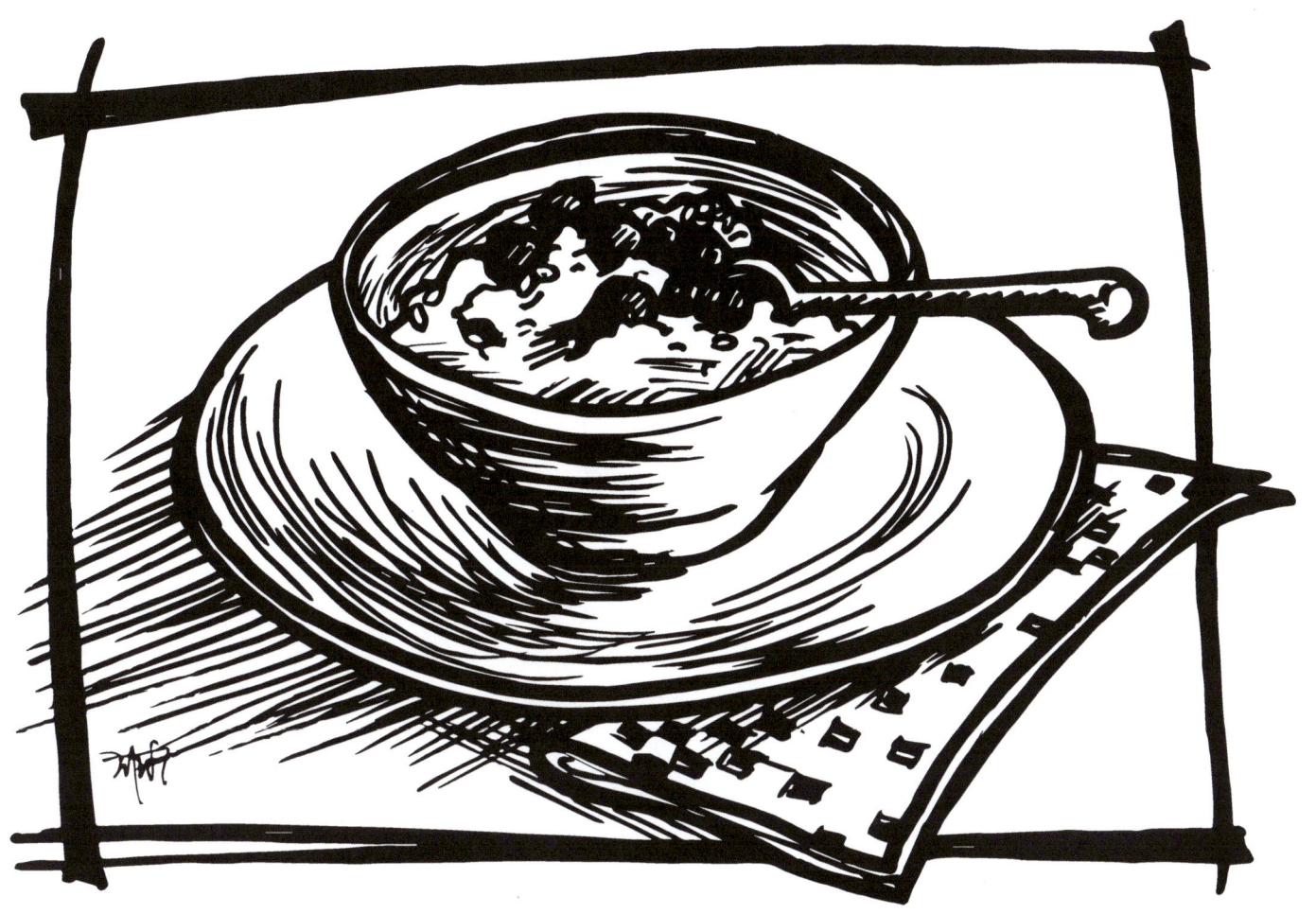

A Word About Cultured Dairy

Cultured dairy products, such as kefir and yogurt, are a beautiful and widely recognized branch of the fermented foods family. I have elected not to write out a specific recipe or "how to" for culturing dairy. I am not well experienced with preparing these foods, but many other folks are. I highly recommend you look to some of these experts, such as those associated with the Weston A. Price Foundation. Try looking on YouTube for lots of good videos, too.

I personally have cultured kefir using raw goat's milk very successfully and easily. However, I did not have great success trying to culture yogurt. Years ago, I made fresh soy milk, and cultured it into yogurt. This was the easiest yogurt recipe ever, once the soy milk was made. More recently, I have made sprouted soy milk, which I would love to make into yogurt one of these days. I do not generally recommend soy products of any kind, except for fermented organic soy, as it is virtually indigestible by humans. However, sprouted soy products can offer variety to those who are intolerant of casein.

Other dairy products which are, or can be cultured include cream cheese, buttermilk, cottage cheese, piima, crème fraiche and numerous traditional products from people groups who have traditionally fermented milk.

www.ingramcontent.com/pod-product-compliance
Lightning Source LLC
Chambersburg PA
CBHW042139290426
44110CB00002B/59